Dermatopathology
Primer of Cutaneous Tumors

Dermatopathology Primer of Cutaneous Tumors

Omar P. Sangueza, MD
Professor of Dermatology
and Pathology
Director of Dermatopathology
Wake Forest University
Health Sciences
Winston-Salem, North Carolina,
USA

Parisa Mansoori, MD
Visiting Fellow in Dermatopathology
Wake Forest University School of Medicine
Winston-Salem, North Carolina, USA

Saleha A. Aldawsari, MD
Visiting Fellow in Dermatopathology
Department of Pathology
Wake Forest University School of Medicine
Winston-Salem, North Carolina, USA

Amir Al-Dabagh, MD
Visiting Fellow in Dermatology
Department of Dermatology
Wake Forest University School of Medicine
Winston-Salem, North Carolina, USA

Sara Moradi Tuchayi, MD, MPH
Research Fellow
Department of Dermatology
Wake Forest University School of Medicine
Winston-Salem, North Carolina,
USA

Amany A Fathaddin, MD
Visiting Fellow in Dermatopathology
Wake Forest University School of Medicine
Winston-Salem, North Carolina, USA

Steven R. Feldman, MD, PhD
Professor of Dermatology and Pathology
Wake Forest University Health Sciences
Winston-Salem, North Carolina, USA

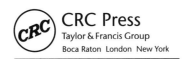

CRC Press
Taylor & Francis Group
Boca Raton London New York

CRC Press is an imprint of the
Taylor & Francis Group, an **informa** business

CRC Press
Taylor & Francis Group
6000 Broken Sound Parkway NW, Suite 300
Boca Raton, FL 33487-2742

© 2016 by Taylor & Francis Group, LLC
CRC Press is an imprint of Taylor & Francis Group, an Informa business

No claim to original U.S. Government works

Printed on acid-free paper
Version Date: 20150527

International Standard Book Number-13: 978-1-4987-0391-8 (Paperback)

Visit the Taylor & Francis Web site at
http://www.taylorandfrancis.com

and the CRC Press Web site at
http://www.crcpress.com

CONTENTS

ACKNOWLEDGEMENTS

The second volume of *Dermatopathology Primer* is a complement to the first volume on inflammatory disease. This volume was produced in collaboration with many of the international fellows of the Section of Dermatopathology of the Wake Forest University School of Medicine.

We want to thank especially Professor Luis Requena from the Department of Dermatology of the Universidad Autonoma de Madrid for allowing us to use some of his wonderful material.

We also thank Mr. Charles P. Sangueza for his help in editing and critically reviewing many chapters of this manuscript.

INTRODUCTION

The second volume of the *Dermatopathology Primer* series deals with neoplastic diseases of the skin. This volume is a complement the first volume on inflammatory diseases.

As we noted in the first volume, the intent of these books is to introduce the basic concepts of dermatopathology to medical students and residents training in pathology and dermatology.

The book is organized into chapters discussing the differentiation of various neoplasms. These include cysts, epidermal, melanocytic lymphoid, and soft tissue neoplasms, both benign and malignant. For each neoplasm we have used illustrations and discussion demonstrating the most characteristic features. In addition, we have also included illustrations of the entities that enter in the differential diagnosis. Because of space limitations and the limited scope of the book, variations of the different neoplasms are not included. For further information the reader is encourage to consult any of several standard books of dermatopathology.

We hope that this book will fulfill the expectations of students beginning the study of dermatopathology.

TUMORS OF THE EPIDERMIS

BENIGN TUMORS • EPIDERMAL PROLIFERATIONS

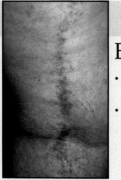

EPIDEMIOLOGY

- Occurs in 1 in 1000 live births
- 80% of lesions appear within the first year of life, with the majority of lesions appearing by age 14. There are rare reports of epidermal nevi appearing in adults
- Mostly sporadic, however, some familial cases have been documented

PATHOPHYSIOLOGY

- Genetic mosaicism is thought to be the underlying cause, likely a postzygotic somatic mutation
- The mutation affects pluripotential cells giving rise to hamartomas of different cell lines

SPECIAL STUDIES

- Extensive epidermal nevi require further work up. These patients require a complete examination, including the eyes, in order to rule out cataracts and optic nerve hypoplasia; and neuroimaging and cardiac studies to rule out aneurysms and patent ductus arteriosus

CLINICAL FEATURES

- The characteristic epidermal nevus presents as a linear, hyperpigmented, papillomatous plaque that can vary from pink to black, velvety to verrucous, flat to thick, and can involve small or extensive areas of the skin
- The lesions are usually asymptomatic
- The inflammatory linear verrucous epidermal nevi (ILVEN) variant is pruritic and may be erythematous or scaly
- The lesions are more common on the trunk or extremities along the Blaschko lines, but may also occur on the face and neck
- Approximately one-third of the patients develop the so-called epidermal nevus syndrome (ENS), an entity in where there is involvement of other systems including the nervous, cardiovascular, urogenital, and/or skeletal

CLINICAL VARIANTS

- The inflammatory linear verrucous epidermal nevi (ILVEN)
- Epidermal nevus syndrome (ENS)

EPIDERMAL NEVUS

INTRODUCTION

Epidermal nevus is a term that encompasses hamartomatous proliferations of epithelium that originate from embryonal ectoderm. They are classified on the basis of the main histologic component: keratinocytes (epidermal nevus), sebaceous gland (nevus sebaceous), pilosebaceous unit (nevus comedonicus), eccrine gland (eccrine nevus), or apocrine gland (apocrine nevus).

HISTOLOGICAL FEATURES

1. Acanthosis
2. Papillomatosis
3. Hyperkeratosis
4. Hyperpigmentation of the basal layer may be seen
5. Thickening of the granular layer

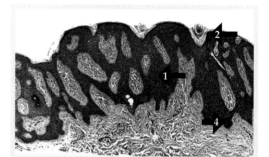

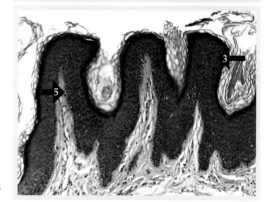

EPIDERMAL NEVUS

HISTOLOGICAL DIFFERENTIAL

1. SEBORRHEIC KERATOSIS:
- Well-circumscribed neoplasm composed of basaloid cells
- Basket weave orthokeratosis
- Horn pseudocysts

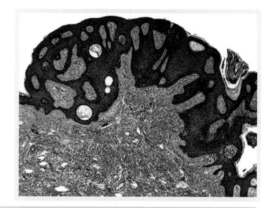

SEBORRHEIC KERATOSIS

IMPORTANT THINGS TO KNOW

- Neoplasms such as basal cell carcinoma (BCC), squamous cell carcinoma (SCC) and keratoacanthoma are not usually associated with epidermal nevi
- Malignancy in epidermal nevus, when it does occur, develops after puberty

Clear cell acanthoma (Degos acanthoma, pale cell acanthoma)

Introduction

Clear cell acanthoma (CCA) is a benign epidermal neoplasm composed of keratinocytes with ample pale cytoplasm and centrally placed nuclei. It consists of a well-demarcated, solitary, shiny, and brown to orange papule or nodule.

Histological features

1. Well-circumscribed lesions composed of uniform pale keratinocytes
2. Distinct transition between the normal epidermis and the paler cells
3. Parakeratosis with variable number of neutrophils
4. Neutrophils are scattered within the acanthoma
5. Absence of granular layer and epidermal melanin
6. Suprapapillary plate thinning, sparing of adnexal epidermis and dilated tortuous dermal blood vessels in the papillary dermis

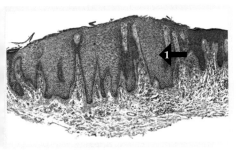 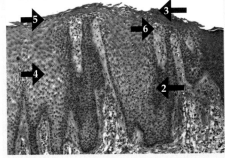

CLEAR CELL ACANTHOMA

Histological differential

1. PSORIASIS VULGARIS:
- No clear cells with distinct transition between the normal epidermis and the clearer/paler cells in the epidermis

2. TRICHILEMMOMA:
- Neutrophils absent
- Outlined by a thick eosinophilic basement membrane
- Peripheral palisading
- Numerous squamous eddies

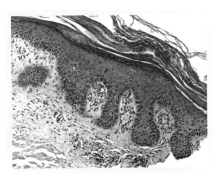 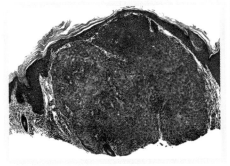

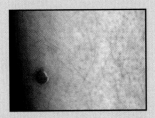

Epidemiology

- Middle-aged; mostly after the age of 40
- Male-to-female ratio is 1:1

Pathophysiology

- It is unclear whether CCA is a true neoplasm or an inflammatory dermatosis

Clinical features

- Solitary, slow-growing, well-demarcated, erythematous to brown papule or nodule with moist eroded surface. In some cases a collarette of scale is present and produces a psoriasiform appearance
- The lesions are asymptomatic and slow growing
- Affects most commonly the legs, but it can be also seen on the thigh, face, forearm, trunk, and inguinal region
- Almost completely blanches with pressure
- Size: 0.3–2 cm (giant clear cell acanthoma >5 cm)

Special studies

- Keratinocytes in the epidermis are glycogen rich and stain with periodic acid-Schiff, diastase labile

---

IMPORTANT THINGS TO KNOW

- The clinical features can be confused with pyogenic granuloma and seborrheic keratosis

Clinical variants

- None

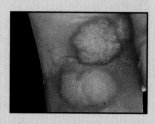

EPIDEMIOLOGY

- Verruca occurs predominantly in children and adolescents although adults are also frequently affected

PATHOPHYSIOLOGY

- Most verrucae vulgaris are induced by HPV-2. Palmoplantar warts are associated with HPV-1 or HPV-4 infection. Verruca plana is associated with HPV-3 and HPV-10
- Epidermodysplasia verruciformis is a rare autosomal recessive genodermatosis due to mutation *EVER1/TMC6 or EVER2/TMC8 genes. Warts induced by different types of HPV*
- In condylomas, HPV-6 and 11 are most commonly identified and are sexually transmitted

CLINICAL FEATURES

- Verruca vulgaris are hard papules found on exposed parts; mostly on the fingers
- Palmoplantar warts are found on the palm or the sole and they are painful
- Verrucae plana are multiple skin-colored or slightly elevated papules on face and extremities
- Condylomas are fleshy exophytic lesion of the anogenital region

SPECIAL STUDIES

- In situ hybridization and immunohistochemistry to subtype HPVs

CLINICAL VARIANTS

- Flat warts (verruca plana)
- Palmoplantar warts (myrmecia warts)
- Condyloma

VIRAL WARTS (VERRUCAE)

INTRODUCTION

Verrucae are lesions caused by human papillomavirus (HPV), which produces various types of warts on different parts of the skin.

HISTOLOGICAL FEATURES

1. Exophytic neoplasm with finger-like projections; compact hyperkeratosis, papillomatosis, hypergranulosis and acanthosis; inward turning of the elongated rete ridges at the edge of the lesion
2. Parakeratosis at the tips of the projections
3. Dilated blood vessels in papillary dermis
4. Large vacuolated cells with small pyknotic nucleus (koilocytes)
- Flat warts or verruca plana show prominent hypergranulosis. The cytoplasm of the cells shows blue-gray inclusions
- Palmoplantar warts or myrmecia warts show red cytoplasmic inclusions
- Epidermodysplasia verruciformis characterized by large cells with conspicuous perinuclear halo. The cytoplasm, which is blue-gray, contains keratohyalin granules

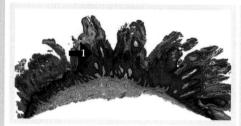

WART 2

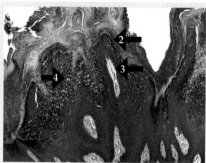

WART 3

HISTOLOGICAL DIFFERENTIAL

- Seborrheic keratosis: horn pseudocysts are seen and basket weave stratum corneum are seen
- Squamous cell carcinoma: atypical pleomorphic cells with mitoses are seen

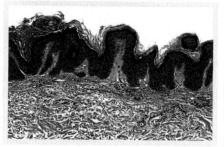

SEBORRHEIC KERATOSIS

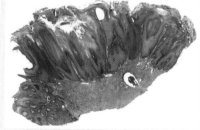

VERRUCOUS SQUAMOUS CELL CARCINOMA

IMPORTANT THINGS TO KNOW

- Patients with epidermodysplasia verruciformis show numerous flat warts

Trichilemmoma (tricholemmoma)

Introduction

Trichilemmoma (tricholemmoma) is a form of benign adnexal neoplasm with differentiation mostly toward the follicular outer root sheath. These lesions are variants of warts and recently it has been demonstrated the presence of papillomavirus DNA in these lesions.

Histological features

1. Small circumscribed and lobular or multilobular proliferation of pale keratinocytes
2. Peripheral palisading of the nuclei
3. Outlined by a thick densely eosinophilic basement membrane
4. Numerous squamous eddies

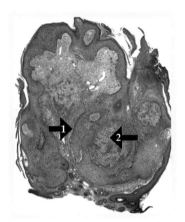 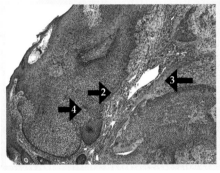

TRICHILEMMOMA

Histological differential

1. Clear cell acanthoma:
- Glycogenated pale segment of epidermis is sharply demarcated from the surrounding skin
- Neutrophils are noted throughout the lesion and in the overlying crust
- Absence of thickening of the basement membrane zone

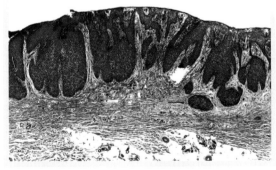

CLEAR CELL ACANTHOMA

Important Things To Know

- Desmoplastic trichilemmoma is characterized by irregular extensions of the outer root sheath which project into sclerotic collagen bundles and may simulate infiltrating squamous cell carcinoma

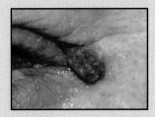

Epidemiology

- The majority of trichilemmoma occur between the age of 20 and 80 years, with a mean age of 30 years
- Male-to-female ratio is approximately 1:1
- Trichilemmoma are not associated with morbidity or mortality

Pathophysiology

- Trichilemmomas are induced by HPV
- A mutation in the tumor suppressor gene *PTEN/MMAC1*, as observed in Cowden syndrome, may play a causative role

Clinical features

- Trichilemmomas appear as simple or multiple small (3–8 mm in diameter) papules or nodules
- Individual lesions may be keratotic or smooth-surfaced and coloration usually matches that of surrounding skin
- Predominantly located on the central face, particularly around the nose and upper lip, but may occur at any non-glabrous site
- Most lesions are clinically misdiagnosed as BCC or benign keratosis
- Multiple trichilemmomas typically present on the facial or genital skin. On genital skin they simulate the clinical pattern of a condyloma, especially if multiple
- Multiple trichilemmomas can be associated with Cowden syndrome (an autosomal dominant condition distinguished by multiple trichilemmoma, sclerotic fibromas, acrokeratosis and adenocarcinoma of the breast, thyroid gland, or gastrointestinal tract)

Special studies

- Hematoxylin and eosin is the stain of choice
- PAS-D (periodic acid-Schiff with diastase) stain may be used to highlight the thickened basement membrane
- A CD34 stain may be used to differentiate between a desmoplastic trichilemmoma and a BCC (CD34 positive in desmoplastic trichilemmoma and negative in BCC)

Clinical Variants

- None

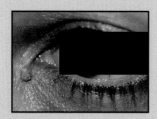

EPIDEMIOLOGY

- Middle-aged to elderly individuals
- Male-to-female ratio is 2:1

PATHOPHYSIOLOGY

- The involved cells are thought to arise from the follicular infundibulum, although the reason for proliferation is unknown

CLINICAL FEATURES

- Solitary, flesh-colored or pink, firm papule which measures from 0.3–1 cm in diameter
- Most commonly found on face (predilection for cheek, upper lip, eyelid)
- Asymptomatic, stable lesions with occasional regression

SPECIAL STUDIES

- In situ hybridization and immunohistochemistry to detect HPV

CLINICAL VARIANTS

- None

INVERTED FOLLICULAR KERATOSIS

INTRODUCTION

Inverted Follicular Keratosis (IFK) is an uncommon benign tumor of the follicular infundibulum that can be confused, both clinically and histologically, with several benign and malignant skin conditions. The lesion typically appears on the face as a solitary firm papule and is characterized histologically by an endophytic proliferation of keratinocytes with the formation of squamous eddies.

HISTOLOGICAL FEATURES

1. Endophytic proliferation of follicular keratinocytes extending downward into the dermis in a well-demarcated, lobular configuration
2. Hyperkeratosis, parakeratosis and occasionally papillomatosis
3. Squamous eddies
4. Mild inflammatory cell infiltrate, predominantly lymphohistiocytic is common in dermis

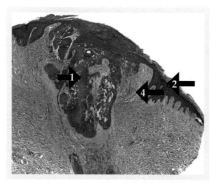
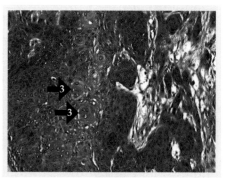

INVERTED FOLLICULAR KERATOSIS

HISTOLOGICAL DIFFERENTIAL

1. SEBORRHEIC KERATOSIS (ESPECIALLY THE IRRITATED VARIANT)
- Seborrheic keratosis are raised above the surrounding skin
- Absence of endophytic component

2. SQUAMOUS CELL CARCINOMA
- SCC is not well demarcated
- Cellular atypia and abnormal mitoses
- Absence of squamous eddies

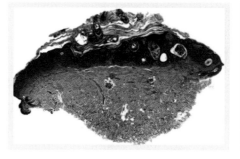
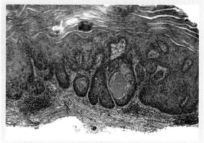

IMPORTANT THINGS TO KNOW

- IFK are essentially warts developing within a hair follicle

Solar lentigo

Introduction

Benign pigmented lesion with an increased number of pigmented keratinocytes.

Histological features

1. Elongation of the rete ridges
2. Basal hyperpigmentation, sometimes quite heavy
3. Solar elastosis is almost always present

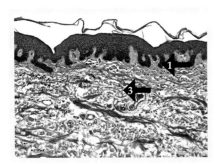 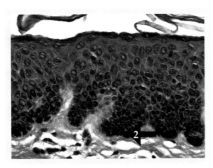

Solar lentigo

Histological differential

1. Lentigo maligna:
- Presence of irregular nests of melanocytes
- Single melanocytes in the upper layers of the epidermis

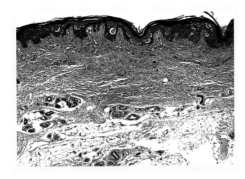

Lentigo maligna

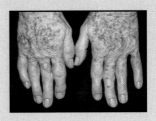

Epidemiology

- Solar lentigo occurs on sun-exposed skin in more than 90% of the white population older than age 60 years, but may be observed in much **younger individuals as well**

Pathophysiology

- It has been suggested that solar lentigo is induced by the mutagenic effect of repeated ultraviolet light exposure
- Carriers of one or two of the melanocortin-1-receptor (*MC1R*) gene variants have a 1.5- to 2-fold increased risk for the development of numerous solar lentigines

Clinical features

- Dark brown to black macules, 3–12 mm or more in diameter; often multiple
- They are distinguished from common freckles by their persistence despite absence of sun exposure

Special studies

- Immunohistochemical analysis: S-100, HMB-45, Melan-A, and tyrosine kinase are negative in the pigmented keratinocytes, but highlight the presence of melanocytes

Clinical Variants

- Hypermelanotic or "ink spot" solar lentigo

Important Things To Know

- Solar lentigos can be very large and simulate melanoma clinically
- Solar lentigo may show transition to reticulated seborrheic keratosis

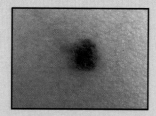

EPIDEMIOLOGY

- Common in elderly
- Increase in number with age
- Sunlight seems to play a role

PATHOPHYSIOLOGY

- Monoclonal in origin, indicating clonal expansion of somatically activating mutations in a specific transmembrane tyrosine kinase receptor, fibroblast growth factor receptor-3

CLINICAL FEATURES

- Sharply defined, tan to black, flat, papular or nodular lesions with a velvety to verrucous surface
- "Stuck-on", waxy appearance
- Usually asymptomatic with minimal pruritis
- Frequently located on sun-exposed areas; trunk, face, upper extremities

SPECIAL STUDIES

- None

CLINICAL VARIANTS

- Dermatosis papulosa nigra
- Stucco keratosis
- Nevoid hyperkeratosis of the nipple
- Oral melanoacanthoma

SEBORRHEIC KERATOSIS

INTRODUCTION

Seborrheic keratoses are the most common benign skin tumor in older individuals characterized by well-demarcated papules with a verrucous surface. They appear "stuck-on" and increase in numbers with age. They are commonly found on the face, neck, and trunk (especially the upper back), as well as the extremities.

HISTOLOGICAL FEATURES

1. Proliferation of basaloid cells with areas of acanthosis and papillomatosis
2. Pseudo-horn cysts
3. Sharp demarcation of the base of the neoplasm
4. Basket weave hyperkeratosis
- Histological variants include **acanthotic, hyperkeratotic, clonal (Borst-Jadassohn appearance), reticulated, irritated and melanoacanthoma variant**

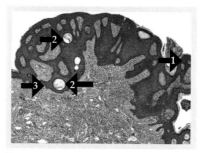
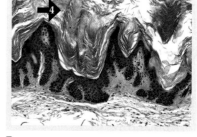

SEBORRHEIC KERATOSIS   PIGMENTED SEBORRHEIC KERATOSIS

HISTOLOGICAL DIFFERENTIAL

1. Epidermal nevus:
- Clinical history is helpful
- Usually lack pseudocysts
2. Squamous cell carcinoma:
- Atypical keratinocytes involving the entire epidermis, dyskeratosis and abundant mitoses

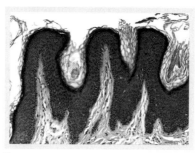
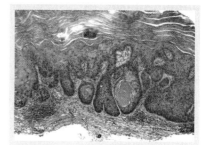

EPIDERMAL NEVUS   SQUAMOUS CELL CARCINOMA

IMPORTANT THINGS TO KNOW

- Leser-Trélat sign is the sudden onset of numerous seborrheic keratoses and may indicate an underlying visceral neoplasm

Warty dyskeratoma

Introduction

Warty dyskeratoma is a benign papulonodular lesion characterized by an endophytic proliferation of squamous epithelium, typically occurring in relation to a folliculosebaceous unit and showing prominent areas of acantholysis.

Histological features

1. Well-demarcated endophytic lesion characterized by prominent acantholytic dyskeratosis
2. Suprabasal clefting with formation of villi
3. Abundant keratin forming a plug within the center of the proliferation
4. Corps rounds and grains, which are dyskeratotic keratinocytes present in the stratum spinosum and granulosum

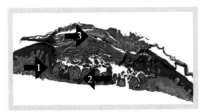

WARTY DYSKERATOMA

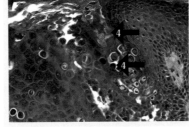

Histological differential

1. Benign familial pemphigus (Hailey–Hailey disease)
- Has more acantholysis
- Acantholysis involving large areas of the epidermis
2. Darier's disease
- Needs clinicopathological correlation
3. Pemphigus vegetans
- Large areas of acantholysis
- Collections of eosinophils in the epidermis

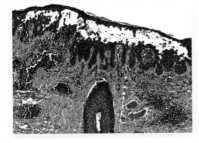

FAMILIAL BENIGN PEMPHIGUS
(HAILEY–HAILEY)

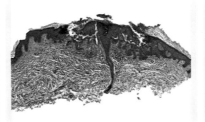

DARIER'S DISEASE

PEMPHIGUS VEGETANS

Epidemiology

- Warty dyskeratoma occurs mostly in middle-aged to elderly adults

Pathophysiology

- There are no known etiological factors

Clinical features

- Most lesions are solitary flesh-colored to brown papules, nodules or cysts with an umbilicated or pore-like center or central keratin plug
- Most are 1–10 mm in size. Occasionally the lesions are multiple
- Most cases asymptomatic but can be pruritic and bleed
- Foul-smelling cheesy discharge possible
- The head and neck region is most commonly involved
- Does not spontaneously regress

Special studies

- Excisional biopsy and immunofluorescent staining to rule out pemphigus vegetans

Important things to know

- The diagnosis is rarely made clinically
- Malignant degeneration has not been associated with warty dyskeratoma
- HPV is not associated despite the warty dyskeratoma

Clinical variants

- None

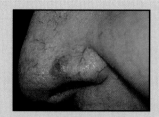

BASAL CELL CARCINOMA AND VARIANTS

INTRODUCTION

Basal cell carcinoma (BCC) is the most common malignant neoplasm in humans. It is destructive locally and has a tendency to recur, but rarely metastasizes. BCC varies in aggressiveness and can be associated with multiple syndromes.

HISTOLOGICAL FEATURES

1. Irregular collections of basaloid cells
2. Neoplastic keratinocytes with large oval basophilic nuclei and scant cytoplasm
3. Clefts between the neoplastic cells and stroma (an artifact produced by the loss of mucin during processing)

Other features:
- Necrotic tumor cells are present among the basaloid cells and sometimes form central pseudocystic spaces filled with mucinous debris

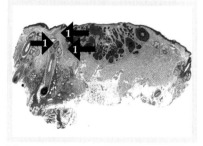

NODULAR BASAL CELL CARCINOMA   BASAL CELL CARCINOMA

HISTOLOGICAL DIFFERENTIAL

1. Squamous cell carcinoma:
- Larger and more eosinophilic cells
- No cleft artifact
- No peripheral palisading
2. Poroma:
- Uniform cellular proliferation of basaloid cells
- Lack necrotic cells
- No clefting
- Lack of stromal changes seen in BCC

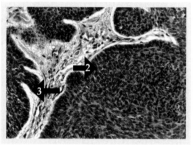

SQUAMOUS CELL CARCINOMA

EPIDEMIOLOGY

- 75% of all diagnosed skin cancers in the United States are BCCs
- Predisposing factors include a history of nonmelanoma skin cancer, Fitzpatrick skin type I and II, prolonged sun exposure in youth, immunosuppression, exposure to arsenic, fiberglass dust, or dry cleaning agents, and previous trauma (smallpox vaccination site, burn scars)
- BCC can be associated with xeroderma pigmentosum (XP), Gorlin's syndrome (basal cell nevus syndrome, BCNS), Bazex syndrome (X-linked dominant condition with features of follicular atrophoderma, multiple BCCs, local anhidrosis, and congenital hypotrichosis) or Rombo syndrome (an autosomal dominant condition distinguished by BCC, atrophoderma vermiculatum, trichoepitheliomas, hypotrichosis, milia, and peripheral vasodilation with cyanosis)

PATHOPHYSIOLOGY

- BCCs develop from keratinocytes in the basal layer (stem cells) of hair follicles, sebaceous glands, and interfollicular basal cells
- A relationship to embryonic closure lines may exist
- The tumor suppressor genes *p53* or *PTCH1* are most commonly mutated
- XP and Gorlin's syndrome have evidence of *PTCH1* mutations

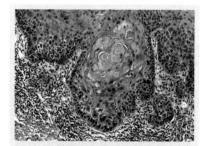 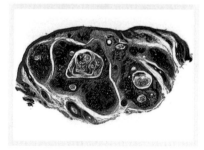

POROMA   TRICHOEPITHELIOMA

CLINICAL VARIANTS

- Nodular
- Superficial (multifocal)
- Morpheaform (infiltrative)
- Fibroepithelioma of Pinkus

BCC VARIANTS

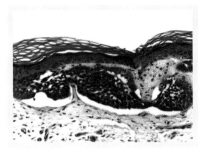

SUPERFICIAL BASAL CELL CARCINOMA

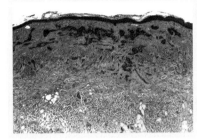

MORPHEAFORM OR INFILTRATIVE
BASAL CELL CARCINOMA

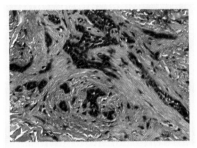

MORPHEAFORM OR INFILTRATIVE
BASAL CELL CARCINOMA

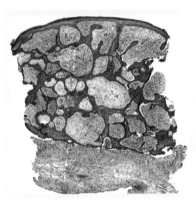

FIBROEPITHELIOMA OF PINKUS

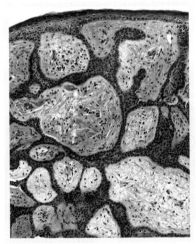

FIBROEPITHELIOMA OF PINKUS

CLINICAL FEATURES

- Pearly red macule, papule, nodule or plaque most common in sun-exposed area especially the nose, face and ears
- Telangiectasia over the neoplasm

SPECIAL STUDIES

- H&E is the stain of choice
- BerEp-4 and cytokeratin 20 to differentiate Merkel cell carcinoma

IMPORTANT THINGS TO KNOW

- Lichen planus like keratosis can mimic BCC clinically

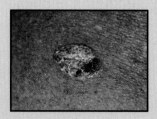

EPIDEMIOLOGY

- It occurs predominantly on sun-exposed skin of older white men, but both sexes are affected
- Invasive carcinoma can develop in up to 8% of untreated cases

PATHOPHYSIOLOGY

- The exact underlying cause remains unclear; however, it is known that chronic sun damage disrupts normal keratinocytic maturation and causes mutation of the tumor suppressor gene mutation (*TP53*)

CLINICAL FEATURES

- The disease presents as an asymptomatic well-defined erythematous scaly plaque

SPECIAL STUDIES

- Immunohistochemical analysis: CK5/6+, HMB-45–, CEA–

BOWEN'S DISEASE

INTRODUCTION

Bowen's disease is a clinical expression of squamous cell carcinoma in situ of the skin.

HISTOLOGICAL FEATURES

1. Full-thickness involvement of epidermis and sometimes the pilosebaceous epithelium by atypical keratinocytes, dyskeratotic cells, and mitoses
2. Loss of the granular layer, parakeratosis, and hyperkeratosis
- Several histological variants have been described: psoriasiform, atrophic, verrucous hyperkeratotic, pigmented and pagetoid variant

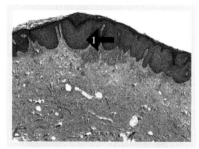
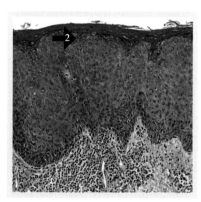

BOWEN DISEASE

HISTOLOGICAL DIFFERENTIAL

1. Bowenoid papulosis:
- Multiple papules on the anogenital areas of young patients
2. Extramammary Paget's disease:
- (CK7+, CEA+)
- Sometimes difficult to distinguish from Pagetoid variant
3. Melanoma in situ
- (S-100+, HMB-45+)
- Sometimes difficult to distinguish from Pagetoid variant

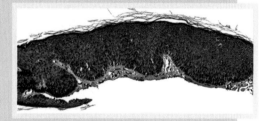

BOWENOID PAPULOSIS

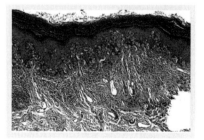

EXTRAMAMMARY PAGET'S DISEASE

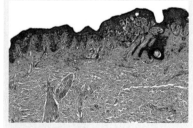

MELANOMA IN SITU

CLINICAL VARIANTS

- Verrucous
- Ulcerated
- Pigmented

IMPORTANT THINGS TO KNOW

- Bowenoid papulosis is indistinguishable from Bowen's disease histologically

KERATOACANTHOMA

INTRODUCTION

Keratoacanthomas are rapidly growing variant of squamous cell carcinomas that may resolve spontaneously leaving an atrophic scar.

HISTOLOGICAL FEATURES

1. Invaginating epidermis with a keratin-filled crater. Adjacent epithelium develops "lips" and shows orthokeratosis, acanthosis, hypergranulosis and parakeratosis
2. Strands of eosinophilic epidermis invade the dermis. Mitoses are present
3. Intraepidermal neutrophilic, eosinophilic microabscesses and horn pearls
4. Involuting lesions begin to take on a flattened, less crateriform appearance. The inflammatory infiltrate becomes largely lichenoid

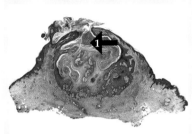

KERATOACANTHOMA

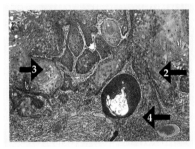

KERATOACANTHOMA

HISTOLOGICAL DIFFERENTIAL

1. Squamous cell carcinoma:
- Intraepidermal microabscesses and tissue eosinophilia are more commonly found in keratoacanthoma
2. Warts:
- Do not show the degree of atypia seen in keratoacanthomas
- Tend to be exophytic

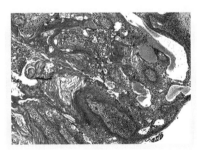

SQUAMOUS CELL CARCINOMA

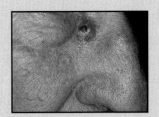

EPIDEMIOLOGY

- Keratoacanthomas develop in the older age groups, particularly in the sixth and seventh decades, and there is a male preponderance

PATHOPHYSIOLOGY

- Exposure to excessive sunlight is the most frequently incriminated factor
- DNA sequences of HPV of both genital and cutaneous types have been detected in up to 55% of keratoacanthomas in immunosuppressed patients

CLINICAL FEATURES

- Solitary pink or flesh-colored dome-shaped nodule with a central keratin plug on the sun-exposed skin. Multiple keratoacanthoma can occur
- It grows rapidly to a size of 1–2 cm, followed by a stationary period. It has a tendency to involute spontaneously, this takes 8–50 weeks. Giant keratoacanthoma is greater than 2 cm and has a predilection for the nose and dorsum of the hand
- Abortive keratoacanthoma is a variant in which involution commences at an early stage
- Keratoacanthoma centrifugum marginatum is a rare variant characterized by progressive peripheral growth with coincident central healing
- Subungual keratoacanthomas grow rapidly; they are more destructive than squamous cell carcinoma in this site

SPECIAL STUDIES

- None

CLINICAL VARIANTS

- Subungual keratoacanthoma is an aggressive carcinoma
- Eruptive keratoacanthomas, which can appear suddenly and in crops

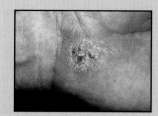

EPIDEMIOLOGY

- SCC occurs in men about two to three times more frequently than it does in women
- Predisposing factors include: Fitzpatrick skin types I and II, being middle-aged or elderly, multiple atypical keratinocytes (AK), a history of nonmelanoma skin cancer, frequent UV light exposure
- SCC is associated with immunosuppressive therapy
- SCC is also associated with chronic skin ulcers, prior X ray treatment, HPV infection, arsenic ingestion, HIV infection, smoking, genetic syndromes such as xeroderma pigmentosum, and toxic exposure to tars and oils

PATHOPHYSIOLOGY

- The primary cause of most SCC is cumulative lifetime UV light exposure; including PUVA
- Inactivation of the tumor suppressor gene *TP53* occurs in up to 90% of all cutaneous SCC lesions. Other tumor suppressor genes found to be mutated include *P16* and *P14*
- Iatrogenic immunosuppression and DNA repair failure, such as in xeroderma pigmentosum, have also been associated with increased incidence of SCC

CLINICAL VARIANTS

- Verrucous
- Keratoacanthoma

SQUAMOUS CELL CARCINOMA

INTRODUCTION

Cutaneous squamous cell carcinoma (SCC) is the second most common cancer of the skin and accounts for 20% of cutaneous malignancies. Most squamous cell carcinomas are readily treated with few sequelae. Larger or more invasive lesions may require aggressive management and have the potential to metastasize.

HISTOLOGICAL FEATURES

Histology will vary based on the different subtypes of SCC, however common features are:
1. Acanthosis
2. Full-thickness intraepidermal proliferation of atypical keratinocytes, cellular atypia and mitoses
3. Atypical keratinocytes in the dermis (the main feature that distinguishes invasive SCC from SCC in situ)
4. Keratinization results in the production of keratin pearls

Other features:
- Hyperkeratosis and parakeratosis
- Atypical keratinocytes may be found in the basal layer and often extend deeply down hair follicles
- Histological variants include: acantholytic, adenoid, spindle cell, clear cell type, signet-ring cell type, verrucous carcinoma, sarcomatoid and pigmented type

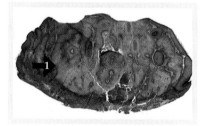

SQUAMOUS CELL CARCINOMA

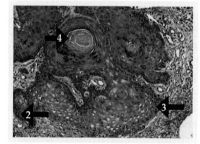

SQUAMOUS CELL CARCINOMA

Histological differential

1. Hypertrophic AK:
- Prominent orthokeratosis with alternating parakeratosis
- Epidermis usually shows irregular psoriasiform hyperplasia and mild papillomatosis
- Atypical keratinocytes are confined to the basal layer
- Presence of vertical collagen bundles and some dilated vessels in the papillary dermis
2. Keratoacanthomatous variant of SCC:
- Exoendophytic lesions with an invaginating mass of keratinizing, well-differentiated squamous epithelium at the sides and bottom of the lesion
- There is a central keratin-filled crater
- Epithelial atypia and mitoses are not a usual features
- There is a mixed infiltrate of inflammatory cells in the adjacent dermis. Eosinophils and neutrophils may be prominent, and these may extend into the epithelial nests to form small microabscesses

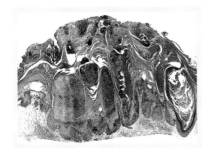

HYPERTROPHIC ATYPICAL
KERATINOCYTES

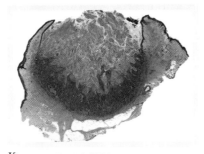

KERATOACANTHOMA

Clinical features
- Hyperkeratotic or ulcerated plaque with a red, inflamed base, a growing tumor, or a non-healing ulcer, often on sun-exposed areas such as the head and neck
- SCC can also occur on the lips, inside the mouth, on the genitalia. It can be de novo or arise from an AK
- SCC is capable of locally infiltrative growth, spread to regional lymph nodes, and distant metastasis, most often to the lung. It is usually asymptomatic unless perineural invasion is present

Special studies
- Immunoperoxidase staining for cytokeratin positivity

Important Things To Know
- If the tumor is poorly differentiated it is associated with a higher risk of metastasis
- Patients who develop one SCC have a 40% risk of developing another SCC within the next 2 years and should be evaluated with a complete skin examination every 6–12 months

MELANOCYTIC NEOPLASMS

BENIGN NEOPLASMS • LENTIGO SIMPLEX (JUVENILE LENTIGO)

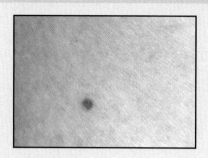

EPIDEMIOLOGY

- The frequency has not been determined
- The most common type of lentigo
- Affects all races and genders

PATHOPHYSIOLOGY

- The etiology is unknown
- Lesions are brown to black freckle-like macules caused by increased melanin production from an increased number of melanocytes in the basal layer

CLINICAL FEATURES

- The lesions are well circumscribed, oval to round, light brown to black macules with regular borders
- They measure only a few millimeters in diameter (usually <5 mm)
- Lentigo simplex can occur anywhere on the body
- The borders are irregular and ill-defined

SPECIAL STUDIES

- Mart-1, Mel-5, and DOPA histochemistry tests can be done to show increased number of melanocytes without nest formation in the basal epidermal layer

INTRODUCTION

Lentigo simplex, is a benign hyperpigmented macule that usually develops at birth or during early childhood that is due to increased melanin production from melanocytes. They are not associated with sun exposure or systemic disease.

HISTOLOGICAL FEATURES

1. Elongation of the rete ridges and increase in number of melanocytes in the basal layer
2. Increased amount of melanin in melanocytes, basal keratinocytes and in the melanophages of the upper dermis

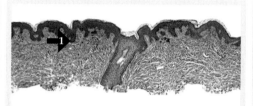

LENTIGO SIMPLEX   LENTIGO SIMPLEX (HIGH POWER)

HISTOLOGICAL DIFFERENTIAL

1. Solar lentigo:
- More significant elongation of the rete ridges, composed of single layers of deeply pigmented basaloid cells and melanocytes
2. Junctional melanocytic nevus:
- Well-circumscribed nevus cell nests either entirely within, or in contact with the lower epidermis

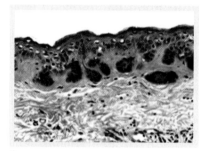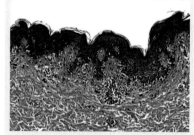

SOLAR LENTIGO   JUNCTIONAL NEVUS

IMPORTANT THINGS TO KNOW

- Multiple lentigines may or may not be associated with numerous autosomal dominant syndromes: LEOPARD syndrome (Lentigines, Electrocardiographic conduction defects, Ocular hypertelorism, Pulmonary stenosis, Abnormalities of genitalis, Retardation of growth and Deafness), Carney complex or NAME/LAMB syndrome (Nevi, Atrial myxoma, Myxoid neurofibroma, Ephelides/Lentigines, Atrial myxoma, Mucocutaneous myxoma, Blue nevi), Peutz-Jeghers syndrome (mucocutaneous lentigines which are present at birth or appear during childhood in combination with intestinal polyposis)

CLINICAL VARIANTS

- None

Melanocytic nevi

Introduction

Melanocytic nevi are common pigmented lesions and can be junctional, compound or intradermal.

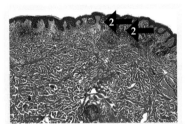

Histological features

1. Junctional nevus: equidistant nests and single melanocytes at the dermal-epidermal junction, regular hyperplasia of the rete ridges. The nevus cells with regular, round to cuboidal, or rarely spindle-shaped appearance
2. Compound nevus: presence of an epidermal and dermal component of nevus, arranged in orderly nests or cords, a gradual decline in the number of nests from the epidermis down to the superficial and reticular dermis, individual nevus cells, dispersed among collagen fiber bundles in the reticular dermis
3. Intradermal nevus: presence of nevus cells only in the dermis

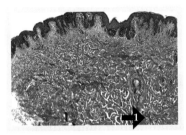

JUNCTIONAL NEVUS

COMPOUND NEVUS

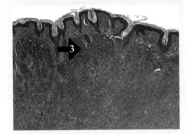

INTRADERMAL NEVUS

Histological differential

Junctional nevus:
1. Lentigo simplex:
- Variable basal hyperpigmentation
- Increased number of single melanocytes in the basal layer
- No nest formation
2. Melanoma in situ:
- Irregular proliferation of nests and single melanocytes in the epidermis
- Single melanocytes can be present in the upper levels of the epidermis

Compound nevus/intradermal nevus:
1. Malignant melanoma:
- Cytological atypia and numerous mitoses in the dermis

Epidemiology

- The prevalence of nevi in the general population is not well documented
- Both sexes are approximately equally affected
- White people have a greater prevalence of nevi than darker-skinned people, and on average have approximately 20 acquired nevomelanocytic nevi
- Acquired melanocytic nevi typically develop before the third decade of life, and begin to disappear thereafter
- Genetic factors play a role in the number of acquired melanocytic nevi

Pathophysiology

- Melanocytic nevi are thought to originate from cells, termed melanoblasts, which migrate from the neural crest to the epidermis

Clinical features

- A round or oval, well-circumscribed, uniformly colored macular lesion with smooth, regular borders
- Color varies from brown to black and their size is always less than 1 cm in diameter
- It may develop anywhere on the body surface
- Compound and intradermal nevi can present as elevated to dome-shaped or polypoid configurations
- Older nevi, predominantly on the trunk, may become pedunculated with time

Special studies

- Hematoxylin and eosin is the stain of choice
- S-100, HMB-45, and Melan-A stain melanocytic lesions

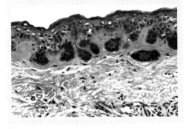

SOLAR LENTIGO

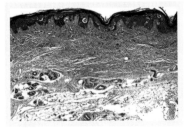

MELANOMA IN SITU

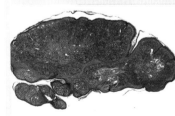

MALIGNANT MELANOMA

Important Things To Know

- Sun exposure promotes the development of melanocytic nevi

Clinical variants

- Unna's
- Miescher
- Clark's
- Spitz nevus
- Reed's nevus
- Blue nevus

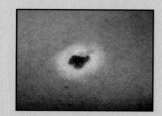

EPIDEMIOLOGY

- Overall incidence of halo nevi in individuals under age 20 is probably <1%
- The majority of halo nevi occur in first 5 decades after birth, with a mean age of approximately 15 years
- Approximately 20% of individuals with halo nevi have vitiligo
- Halo nevi are equally common in all races and both sexes

PATHOPHYSIOLOGY

- Pathophysiology is not completely understood, although both cellular and humoral immunological factors are implicated
- Depigmentation of the central nevus is believed to result from the immunologically mediated destruction of nevus cells by CD8+ T cells
- Depigmentation of the halo area may result from the destruction of melanocytes secondary to the diffusion of an unknown cytotoxic factor

CLINICAL FEATURES

- The central nevus typically is 3–6 mm in diameter, has homogeneous coloration, and is well circumscribed
- The depigmented halo measures in width from a few millimeters to several centimeters and is usually symmetric
- Predominantly located on the back, but may be found in any location
- 25–50% of affected individuals have multiple halo nevi

SPECIAL STUDIES

- Melan-A/MART-1 stain can be used to identify any residual melanocytes

CLINICAL VARIANTS

- None

HALO NEVUS (SUTTON'S NEVUS)

INTRODUCTION

Halo nevi are melanocytic nevi surrounded by a zone of depigmentation or halo of leukoderma. The onset of the ring of depigmentation occurs over several weeks to months. These lesions are more common in children and young adults. In most cases, the central nevus undergoes involution, with subsequent re-pigmentation of the area of depigmentation.

HISTOLOGICAL FEATURES

1. The central nevus may be compound, junctional or dermal
2. A dense band-like inflammatory infiltrate of the papillary dermis, in early stages, in which lymphocytes and histiocytes predominate

Other features:
- At later stages, few, if any, distinct nevus cells can be identified
- Decrease or total absence of melanocytes and increase in Langerhans cells in depigmented zone

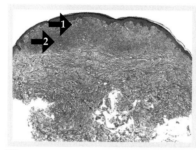

HISTOPATHOLOGY OF HALO NEVUS

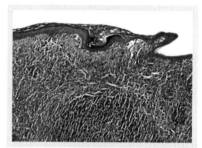

HALO NEVUS HIGH POWER HIGHLIGHTED PROMINENT MELANOCYTES AND LYMPHOCYTES

HISTOLOGICAL DIFFERENTIAL

1. Melanoma:
- Patchy inflammatory infiltrate, more prominent on the periphery
- Increased cellularity
- Mitosis may be found
- No maturation with progressive descend

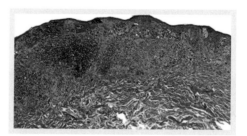

MALIGNANT MELANOMA

IMPORTANT THINGS TO KNOW

- Halo nevi are believed to be an immunologic reaction to a nevus
- The presence of one or more halo nevi may indicate incipient vitiligo
- Early lesion of halo nevi can mimic melanoma and biopsy may be required for the proper diagnosis

Spitz nevus

Introduction

A Spitz nevus is a type of melanocytic nevus which is usually found in children and young adults.

Histological features

1. Nests of large epithelioid cells and/or spindle cells extending in a wedge configuration from the epidermis to the reticular dermis
2. Maturation with progressive descend, with larger cells near the epidermis and smaller cells at the base
3. The large epithelioid and spindle cells have an abundant amphophilic cytoplasm, open chromatin, little, if any, melanin pigment, and prominent eosinophilic or amphophilic nucleoli
4. Epidermal hyperplasia with acanthosis, papillomatosis and hyperkeratosis
5. Clefts between the epidermal and the melanocytic component
6. Kamino bodies that contain basement membrane material are usually found at dermoepidermal junction
- Pigmented spindle cell of Reed is characterized by prominent melanin pigment in addition to other features
- Intraepidermal Spitz nevus is characterized by a proliferation of epithelioid melanocytes in the epidermis without a dermal component
- Intradermal Spitz nevus is characterized by the presence of epithelioid melanocytes in the dermis without an epidermal component

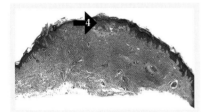

Spitz nevus

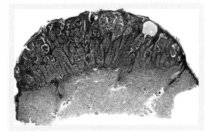

Spitz nevus

Histological differential

1. Melanoma:
- The lesions are asymmetric
- Poorly circumscribed
- No maturation with progressive descend
- Mitotic figures in the deeper areas of the lesion
- Single melanocytes at all levels of the epidermis
- No epidermal hyperplasia

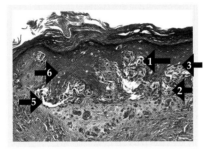

Spitzoid melanoma

Important Things To Know

- It is advised that small Spitz nevi be completely excised as a precaution since differentiation from melanoma is often difficult
- Recurrences rates after the incomplete excision of a Spitz nevus range from 7–16%
- Although benign, melanocyte nests from a Spitz nevus may disseminate to lymph nodes

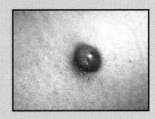

Epidemiology

- The prevalence of Spitz nevi in the general population of Australia is 1.4 per 100,000
- The majority of Spitz nevi are acquired after birth, but up to 7% are estimated to be congenital in origin
- Spitz nevi occur in all age groups, with one-third of cases in individuals less than 10 years, one-third between 10 and 20 years, and one-third over 20 years of age
- However, they are rare in individuals over the age of 40 and are predominantly found in light-skinned individuals
- Both sexes are approximately equally affected

Pathophysiology

- The pathophysiology of Spitz nevi is greatly unknown, and the majority of them have no known precipitated cause
- The widespread onset of Spitz nevi have been linked with HIV infection, chemotherapy, Addison's disease, pregnancy, puberty, and trauma
- The association with pregnancy and puberty indicates a possible hormonal causation

Clinical features

- A dome-shaped, well-circumscribed, hairless papule or nodule often accompanied by telangiectasia
- The color varies from pink to tan and their size is ranges in diameter from 2 mm to 2 cm. In 95% of patients, the nevus is less than 1 cm in diameter
- They are predominantly found on the head and neck area, although they may be found on any part of the body
- Multiple Spitz nevi may arise in a disseminated or agminated pattern

Special studies

- Hematoxylin and eosin is the stain of choice
- S-100, HMB-45, and Melan-A stain melanocytic lesions

Clinical Variants

- Agminated

Spitz nevus variants

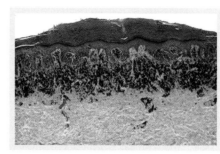

Pigmented spindle cell of Reed

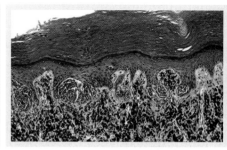

Pigmented spindle cell of Reed

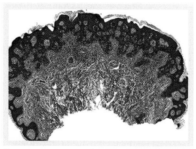

Intraepidermal Spitz nevus

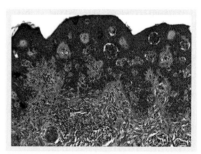

Intraepidermal Spitz nevus

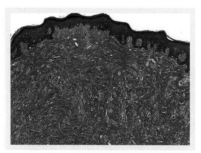

Intradermal Spitz nevus

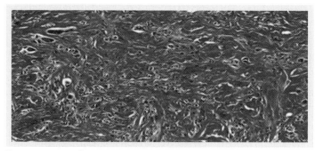

Intradermal Spitz nevus

Blue nevus

Introduction

Blue nevus (BN) is a benign, usually intradermal, melanocytic lesion characterized by pigmented dendritic spindle-shaped melanocytes and more rarely, epithelioid melanocytes. The melanocytes are usually separated by thickened collagen bundles.

Histological features

1. Pigmented spindle-shaped melanocytes
2. Thickened collagen bundles in mid and upper dermis

Epithelioid blue nevus:
- Dermal aggregates of round to oval melanocytes
- Centrally placed nuclei (fried egg appearance)
- Coarse granules of melanin in their cytoplasm

Deep penetrating nevus:
- Vertically oriented neoplasm
- Epithelioid and spindle melanocytes in the dermis
- Epithelioid melanocytes can have spitzoid features
- Melanocytes can be present around adnexal structures

Combined blue nevus:
- Blue nevus with overlying junctional, compound or intradermal nevus

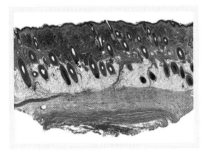
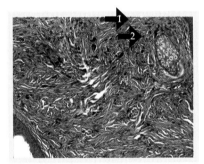

BLUE NEVUS

Histological differential

1. Desmoplastic melanoma:
- Proliferation of spindle cells with variable degree of atypia in the dermis
- Patchy infiltrates of lymphocytes
- In some cases there is an epidermal component
2. Tumoral melanosis:
- These are lesion in which there are only melanophages in the dermis
- The melanophages are loaded with coarse granules of melanin

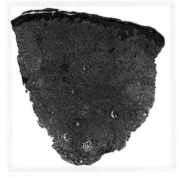
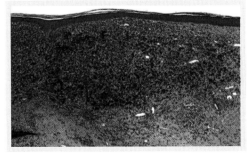

TUMORAL MELANOSIS

DESMOLASTIC MELANOMA

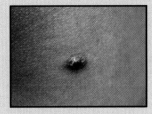

Epidemiology

- BN is relatively frequent, has predilection for females
- Presents mainly in young adults between the second and fourth decades
- Although most tumors are acquired, congenital examples have been documented
- Familial cases may be seen and usually present with multiple lesions

Pathophysiology

- Blue nevi represent benign tumors of dermal melanocytes
- In general, melanocytes disappear from the dermis during the second half of gestation, but some residual melanin-producing cells remain in the scalp, sacral region, and dorsal aspect of the distal extremities
- Somatic activating mutations in *GNA11* and *GNAQ* (primarily the latter) have been detected in 65–75% of blue nevi

Clinical features

- The most common presentation consists of a single asymptomatic, relatively well-circumscribed, dome-shaped blue or blue-black papule less than 1 cm in diameter
- The characteristic blue color is produced by the Tyndall effect
- Tumors may rarely present as a plaque
- Eruptive lesions have rarely been documented
- The anatomical distribution is wide, but most lesions occur on the distal upper limbs (particularly the dorsum of the hand), followed by the lower limbs, scalp, face and buttocks

Clinical variants

- Speckled BN
- Hypopigmented BN
- Widespread BN

SPECIAL STUDIES

- Diffusely positive for melanocytic markers including S-100, HMB-45, Melan-A and microphthalmia transcription factor (MITF-1)

BLUE NEVUS VARIANTS

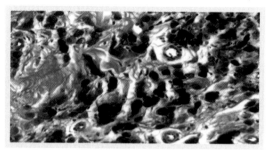

EPITHELIOID BLUE NEVUS

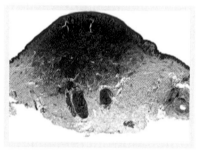

DEEP PENETRATING NEVUS

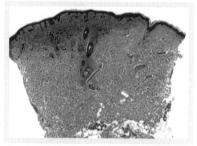

COMBINED NEVUS

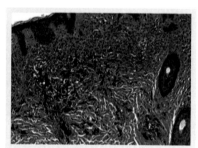

COMBINED NEVUS

IMPORTANT THINGS TO KNOW

- Tyndall effect explains the blue clinical appearance due to deep dermal deposits of melanin which absorbs longer wavelengths of light (red) and reflects shorter wave lengths (blue)

INTRODUCTION

Malignant melanoma (MM) is a skin cancer of the melanocytes, the pigment-producing cells of the skin. It has the ability to metastasize to any organ in the body, especially the brain and heart.

HISTOLOGICAL FEATURES

- Melanomas in situ (MIS)
1. Proliferation of irregular nests with areas of confluence and single melanocytes in epidermis
2. Single melanocytes at different levels of the epidermis including the stratum corneum

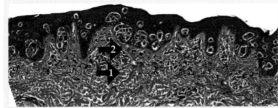

MELANOMA IN SITU

INVASIVE MELANOMA

Other features:
- In some cases, melanocytes replace completely the basal layer of the epidermis
- Solar elastosis; when melanomas developed in sun-exposed areas (lentigo maligna)

- Invasive melanomas
1. Atypical melanocytes in the dermis

Other features:
- Neoplastic cells can form nodules (nodular melanoma)

Acral-lentiginous and mucosal melanoma:
- Presence of dendritic melanocytes
- Containing coarse granules of melanin A
- Extension into the upper levels of the epidermis

Desmoplastic or neurotropic melanoma:
- Proliferation of spindle cells within the dermis
- Minimal atypia
- Resemble other spindle cell proliferations including scars
- One characteristic feature is the presence of lymphoid aggregates
- An epidermal component may or may not be present

There are many other types of melanomas:
a. Amelanotic melanomas
b. Nevoid melanomas
c. Melanoma simulating Spitz nevus (spitzoid melanoma)
d. Melanoma with small nevus-like cells (small cell melanoma)
e. Clear cell sarcoma: melanoma of soft parts

HISTOLOGICAL DIFFERENTIAL

1. Spitz nevus:
- Symmetric lesion
- Spindle and/or epithelioid melanocytes which mature with progressive descend
- Epidermal hyperplasia
- Kamino bodies
- Clefts between the epidermal and melanocytic component
2. Mammary and extramammary Paget's disease:
- Melanoma in situ needs to be differentiated from
- In MIS atypical melanocytes replaced the basal layer, which is spared in Paget's disease

31

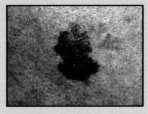

EPIDEMIOLOGY

- Risk factors: fair skin, history of sunburns, more than 50 moles, atypical moles, close relative who had melanoma
- Only 4% of all skin cancers are MM, but MM makes up the majority (74%) of skin cancer-related deaths worldwide. However, low risk melanoma patients (Breslow's thickness <1 mm) have a 90% cure rate when the cancer is found early and appropriately excised
- It is the sixth most common cancer in the United States
- Current lifetime risk is 1 per 60 Americans for invasive MM in 2008, 1 per 32 Americans if noninvasive MM is included
- Highest incidence is in Australia and New Zealand:
  o Australia and New Zealand incidence in 2002: 37.7 per 100,000 men and 29.4 per 100,000 women
  o North America incidence in 2002: 6.4 per 100,000 men and 11.7 per 100,000 women

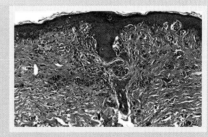

SPITZ NEVUS

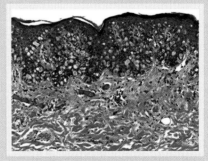

PAGET'S DISEASE

Pathophysiology

- There are both genetic and environmental factors that play a role in the development of MM
- The genetic factors involved in development of melanoma are mutations in chromosome 9p21.25, cyclin-dependent kinase inhibitor 2A (CDKN2A) and cyclin-dependent kinase 4 (CDK4). All are tumor suppressor genes
- The environmental factors correlated with MM are intense periods of sun exposure and living at higher elevations in closer proximity to the sun

Clinical features

- ABCDEs of diagnosing melanoma (Asymmetry – one side unlike the other; Border – irregular, scalloped or poorly defined border; Color – variation in color within the lesion including shades of tan, brown, black, white, red or blue; Diameter – often melanoma lesions are 6 mm in diameter when diagnosed, but can be smaller or larger; Evolution/Elevation/Enlargement – any mole or skin lesion that changes size, shape or color should be evaluated for melanoma)
- Can occur anywhere on the skin, nails and mucosae, regardless if sun exposed, but most commonly occurs on the backs, arms of men, and legs of women
- Can appear on previously normal skin or moles

Special studies

- Primary cutaneous melanoma is can be seen in hematoxylin and eosin sections
- Melanomas are positive for S-100, Melan-A, pan-melanoma and HMB-45 positive
- Desmoplastic melanomas are S-100 positive but negative for Melan-A and HMB-45

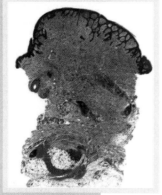

Desmoplastic melanoma

Clinical Variants

- Melanomas in sun-exposed skin
- Melanomas in skin not exposed to sun
- Acral melanomas
- Mucosal melanomas

Melanoma variants

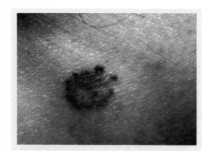

Melanoma of back

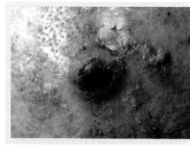

Nodular melanoma

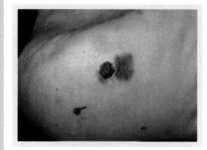

Acral melanoma

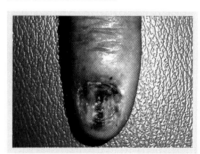

Subungual melanoma

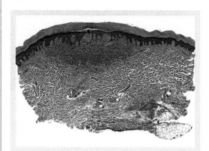

Acral Melanoma

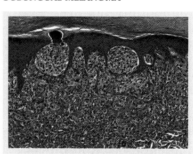

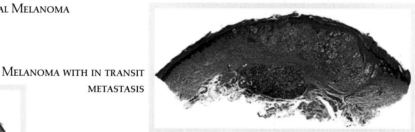

Melanoma with in transit metastasis

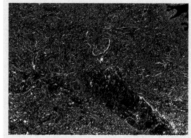

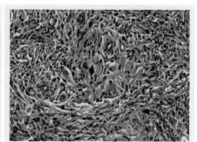

Important Things To Know

- Tumor thickness is the best prognostic marker
- The presence of metastases indicates a poor prognosis; the long-term survival rate is only 5%
- Acral-lentiginous melanoma (ALM) accounts for 5–10% of primary cutaneous MMs and most common melanoma in Asians (up to 45%) and in blacks (up to 70%). Occur on the soles, palms, fingernail or toenail beds

TUMORS OF CUTANEOUS APPENDAGES

HAIR FOLLICLE TUMORS • TRICHOEPITHELIOMA

INTRODUCTION

Desmoplastic trichoepithelioma is a histological variant of trichoepitheliomas with extensive stromal sclerosis (desmoplasia); it occurs almost always on the face.

Trichoepitheliomas are benign tumors derived from the hair follicle. Some regard it as a distinct variant of trichoblastoma.

HISTOLOGICAL FEATURES

1. Well-circumscribed neoplasm
2. Collections of uniform basaloid cells in reticulate or cribriform pattern
3. Stromal clefts
4. No retraction artifact between the neoplastic cells and the stroma
5. Papillary mesenchymal bodies
6. Horn cysts and calcification
7. Fibrous stroma

Desmoplastic trichoepithelioma:
- Composed of cords and strands of basaloid cells with hyperchromatic nuclei and small amounts of cytoplasm
- The neoplastic cells are surrounded by a characteristic rim of collagen
- Prominent fibrotic stroma
- Calcification and foreign body granulomas
- Tadpole- or comma-shaped epithelial projections (paisley-tie pattern)

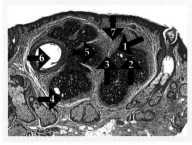

TRICHOEPITHELIOMA

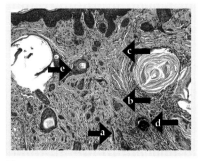

DESMOPLASTIC TRICHOEPITHELIOMA

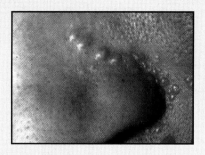

EPIDEMIOLOGY

- Appear around puberty

PATHOPHYSIOLOGY

- It is regarded as poorly differentiated hamartomas of the hair germ
- Multiple familial trichoepitheliomas have an autosomal dominant mode of inheritance due to a mutation in the *CYLD* gene

CLINICAL FEATURES

- Three distinct types: solitary, multiple, and desmoplastic
  - Solitary and multiple have identical histological features
  - Desmoplastic is a distinct entity and will be discussed separately

Solitary trichoepithelioma:
- Small, skin-colored papules on the face, especially around the nose, upper lip, and cheeks. Occasionally develop on the trunk, neck, scalp, and lower extremities

Multiple trichoepithelioma (epithelioma adenoids cysticum):
- Numerous, small papules distributed on the face, usually around the nasolabial folds, forehead, chin, and preauricular area; lesions may coalesce to form plaques and nodules
- Typical onset in childhood or puberty
- Usually inherited in autosomal dominant fashion but may occur sporadically
- Benign, but there are documented cases of basal cell carcinoma (BCC) development in trichoepithelioma
- The Brooke-Spiegler syndrome is the association of multiple trichoepitheliomas with cylindromas and/or spiradenomas

Desmoplastic trichoepithelioma:
- More common in women and young adults
- Types: solitary familial desmoplastic trichoepithelioma, multiple familial, and non-familial tumors
- Usually present as asymptomatic, firm, solitary hard annular lesion with raised border and depressed center
- Do not grow more than 1 cm in diameter; benign with no risk for development of carcinoma

SPECIAL STUDIES

- Immunohistochemical staining: strong reactions for keratins (CK) 5/6 and CK8

HISTOLOGICAL DIFFERENTIAL

1. Syringoma:
- Composed of cords, strands and collections of cells embedded in a sclerotic stroma
- The cells are larger and have an eosinophilic cytoplasm
- No horn cysts, foreign body granulomas or calcification
- Cells contain carcinoembryonic antigen (CEA) but not involucrin
- Usually multiple and periorbital
2. Basal cell carcinoma:
- Is asymmetrical
- Irregular collections of basaloid cells
- Horn cysts, calcification, and papillary mesenchymal bodies are rare
- Clefts between epithelium and stroma

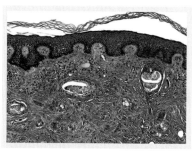

SYRINGOMA

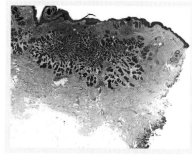

BASAL CELL CARCINOMA

CLINICAL VARIANTS

- Solitary
- Multiple
- Desmoplastic

TRICHOBLASTOMA

INTRODUCTION

Trichoblastoma is a benign tumor with mostly follicular germinative differentiation. It is likely to be on a spectrum with trichoepithelioma (also called immature, solitary, and giant trichoepithelioma).

HISTOLOGICAL FEATURES

1. Circumscribed dermal tumor with no epidermal connections
2. Peripheral palisading of nuclei
3. Follicular differentiation resembling hair bulbs and papillae
4. Fibrotic stroma
5. Clefts in the stroma

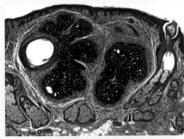
TRICHOBLASTOMA

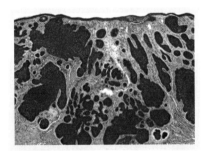
TRICHOBLASTOMA

HISTOLOGICAL DIFFERENTIAL

1. Trichoepithelioma:
• Smaller and more superficial than trichoblastoma
2. Basal cell carcinoma:
• Cleft between epithelium and stroma
• Myxoid stroma

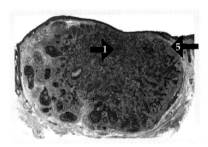
TRICHOEPITHELIOMA

BASAL CELL CARCINOMA

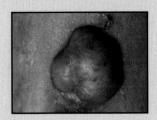

EPIDEMIOLOGY

• Adults
• Affects males and females equally

PATHOPHYSIOLOGY

• It is constituted largely of follicular germinative cells

CLINICAL FEATURES

• Slow-growing, solitary, large (>1 cm) nodule in the deep dermis and subcutis
• Any location, especially scalp, face, trunk, and genital area
• Usually does not involve distal extremities

SPECIAL STUDIES

• CK7, CK8, and CK19 expressed

IMPORTANT THINGS TO KNOW
• Associated with nevus sebaceous

CLINICAL VARIANTS
• None

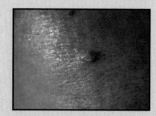

EPIDEMIOLOGY

- Mostly occurring during adulthood
- No sex predilection

PATHOPHYSIOLOGY

- It is a follicularly differentiated hamartoma

CLINICAL FEATURES

- Usually presents as a solitary papule or nodule on the face, scalp, or sometimes the upper trunk; about 0.5 cm in diameter
- May be centrally umbilicated, with tuft of fine hairs emanating from it
- Clinically, may be confused with a BCC or nevus

SPECIAL STUDIES

- None

CLINICAL VARIANTS

- None

TRICHOFOLLICULOMA

INTRODUCTION

Trichofolliculomas are rare pilar tumors.

HISTOLOGICAL FEATURES

1. One or several dilated follicles from which many miniaturized hair follicles radiate with different degrees of differentiation
2. Central follicle opens up on surface, with keratinous material and sometimes villous hairs
3. Follicles branching to secondary or tertiary follicles
4. Relative cellular connective tissue stroma

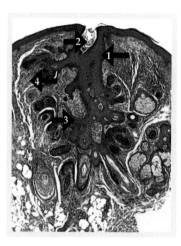
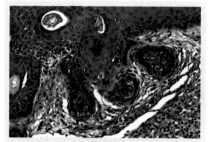

TRICHOFOLLICULOMA

HISTOLOGICAL DIFFERENTIAL

1. Dilated pore of Winer:
- Instead of small hair follicles, there are finger-like epithelial projections that radiate into the surrounding dermis
2. Pilar sheath acanthoma:
- Similar to dilated pore of Winer, but with collections of thick acanthotic epithelium

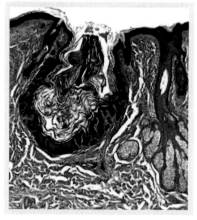
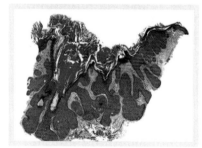

PILAR SHEATH ACANTHOMA

DILATED PORE OF WINER

IMPORTANT THINGS TO KNOW

- There is a variant of trichofolliculoma in which large sebaceous follicles connect to a central cavity or sinus termed sebaceous trichofolliculoma also known as folliculosebaceous cystic hamartoma

Pilar sheath acanthoma

Introduction

Pilar sheath acanthoma (PSA) is a benign adnexal neoplasm. Clinically, it resembles a comedo with a central keratotic plug. Histologically, it has a dilated infundibulum lined by prominent acanthotic epithelium composed of cells with an eosinophilic cytoplasm.

Histological features

1. Central infundibular cystic cavity opening to the epidermal surface and extending down into lower dermis
2. Cyst filled with soft keratinaceous material
3. The cyst wall composed of an acanthotic lobular epithelium forming buds. Cells with ample eosinophilic cytoplasm and centrally placed nuclei resemble the isthmus of the hair follicle

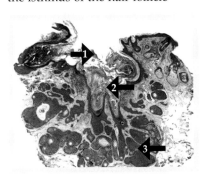

Pilar sheath acanthoma

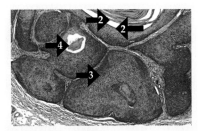

Pilar sheath acanthoma

Histological differential

1. Dilated pore of Winer:
- Larger opening of cystic cavity to epidermal surface
- The cells of the epithelium lining the cystic wall resemble the infundibulum of the hair follicle. The collections of cells are also less prominent
- Foci of keratinization of lobular buds not seen
2. Trichofolliculoma:
- Radiation of small hair follicles from the wall of the central cyst
- Occasional presence of fine, colorless hair
- Prominent fibrovascular stroma not seen in PSA

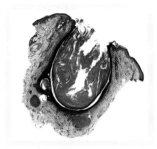

Dilated pore of Winer
Trichofolliculoma

Important Things To Know

- No malignant potential for PSA has been documented and further treatment is unnecessary
- PSA is not associated with a systemic disease

Epidemiology

- Rare follicular hamartoma occurring in middle-aged to elderly individuals
- No gender predilection

Pathophysiology

- It is a follicular neoplasm differentiated toward the infundibulum and the isthmus

Clinical features

- Solitary, flesh-colored papule or nodule with small central depression and keratotic plug
- Most commonly occurs on skin of the upper lip

Special studies

- None

Clinical variants

- None

EPIDEMIOLOGY

- Rare condition with relative frequency of 3 to 10 per 100,000
- Most often affects middle-aged or elderly patients with female predominance

PATHOPHYSIOLOGY

- TFI is thought to originate from the infundibulum with differentiation toward the isthmus cells, although the reason for the proliferation is unknown

CLINICAL FEATURES

- Solitary, flesh-colored or sometimes hypopigmented macule, thin papule or plaque
- Sometimes they may appear slightly atrophic
- Predilection for face and scalp
- Often diagnosed incidentally upon excision of other tumors
- TFI may occur in an eruptive fashion

SPECIAL STUDIES

- None

CLINICAL VARIANTS

- Solitary
- Multiple or eruptive

TUMOR OF THE FOLLICULAR INFUNDIBULUM

INTRODUCTION

Tumor of the follicular infundibulum (TFI) is an uncommon benign adnexal neoplasm. It is a nonspecific lesion seen in middle-aged or older individuals, and often occurs on the face or scalp. The characteristic histopathological feature is a subepidermal plate-like proliferation.

HISTOLOGICAL FEATURES

1. Horizontal plate-like proliferation of pale, isthmic keratinocytes in the superficial dermis
2. Reticulate structure with multiple connections to the overlying epidermis
3. Sharp demarcation of the lateral edges of the lesion with peripheral palisading

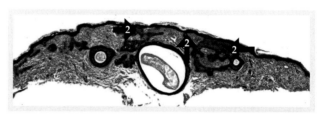

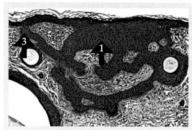

TUMOR OF THE
FOLLICULAR
INFUNDIBULUM

HISTOLOGICAL DIFFERENTIAL

1. Basal cell carcinoma:
- Composed of basaloid cells with large nuclei and small amounts of cytoplasm
- BCC does not form a plate-like proliferation in the dermis
- BER-EP4 is positive
2. Trichilemmoma:
- Characterized by an exophytic nodular proliferation of cells with a pale cytoplasm
- Squamous eddies present in variable amounts

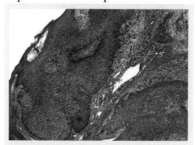

TRICHILEMMOMA

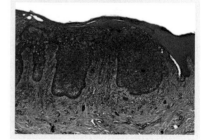

BASAL CELL CARCINOMA

IMPORTANT THINGS TO KNOW

- TFI can be clinically confused with basal cell carcinoma

Sebaceous hyperplasia

Introduction

Sebaceous hyperplasia is a common, benign and asymptomatic condition of sebaceous glands in adults of middle-aged or older. There is no known potential for malignant transformation.

Histological features

1. Enlarged sebaceous gland with multiple mature sebaceous lobules or acini
2. Lobules having one or more basal cell layers

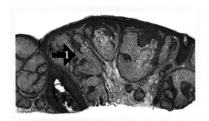
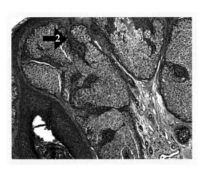

Sebaceous hyperplasia

Histological differential

1. Nevus sebaceous:
- Lobules are aberrant
- Ducts open into the epidermis
- Epidermal hyperplasia
- In some cases presence of apocrine glands, trichoblastomas and syringocystadenoma papilliferum
2. Sebaceous adenoma:
- More than two cell layers of germinative epithelium

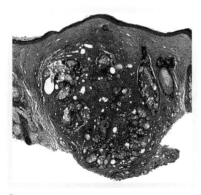

Nevus sebaceous

Sebaceous adenoma

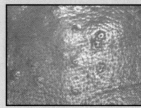

Epidemiology

- Common in aging adults, reported to occur in approximately 1% of the healthy population and 25% of the population over age 30
- There is no relationship between the skin type and the occurrence of these lesions
- There is a higher prevalence of sebaceous hyperplasia in transplant patients
- The difference in prevalence between sexes is unknown

Pathophysiology

- The etiology remains unclear
- A decrease in the circulating levels of androgen associated with aging is thought to be an underlying cause
- Postulated cofactors include ultraviolet radiation and long-term immunosuppression

Clinical features

- One or more whitish-yellow or skin-colored papules that are soft and vary in size from 2–9 mm
- Often asymptomatic, commonly found on the central and upper face
- Occasionally they are also located on the chest, upper arms, areola, oral mucosa, and vulva
- These papules have a central umbilication that corresponds to a central follicular infundibular ostium
- Some papules may have telangiectasias
- Beaded lines represent a unique expression of sebaceous gland hyperplasia in which a linear array of hyperplastic sebaceous glands is present in the vicinity of the clavicle or on the neck
- Biopsy is occasionally indicated to exclude BCC

Special studies

- None

Important Things To Know

- Dermoscopy may be useful in the clinical diagnosis of nodular basal cell carcinoma versus sebaceous hyperplasia
- Dermoscopy shows a haphazard distribution of vessels on the surface of basal cell carcinoma, whereas the vessels in sebaceous hyperplasia occur only in the valleys between the small yellow lobules

Clinical Variants

- None

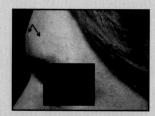

EPIDEMIOLOGY

- Tends to occur in individuals >40 years of age
- Both genders seem to be affected equally with a slight predilection for women

PATHOPHYSIOLOGY

- It is a neoplasm composed of immature sebaceous cells admixed with scattered mature sebocytes
- Some lesions are associated with Muir-Torre syndrome

CLINICAL FEATURES

- Solitary yellow or orange, smooth-surfaced papule or nodule with rolled borders
- Anatomic site: face, scalp, and neck
- Slowly growing, usually asymptomatic and <1 cm in diameter
- Ulceration and bleeding may occur
- Association with Muir-Torre syndrome (characterized also by multiple kerato-acanthomas and visceral carcinomas, especially colonic adenocarcinoma)

SPECIAL STUDIES

- No histologic features of sebaceoma could reliably pinpoint the association of Muir-Torre syndrome, but loss of nuclear staining for MLH-1 or MSH-2 suggests microsatellite instability

CLINICAL VARIANTS

- None

SEBACEOMA

INTRODUCTION

Sebaceomas are distinctive benign neoplasms of adnexal epithelium histologically differentiating toward sebaceous cells. Clinically, these tumors present as yellow to orange papules or nodules on the face or scalp of older individuals and can be associated with the Muir-Torre syndrome.

HISTOLOGICAL FEATURES

1. Symmetric, well-circumscribed lesions composed of lobules with smooth borders localized in the dermis which may extend into the subcutaneous fat
2. Individual lobules show an admixture of basaloid cells or seboblasts and small clusters of mature sebaceous cells
3. Seboblasts predominate in sebaceoma and mature sebaceous cells may be present only focally

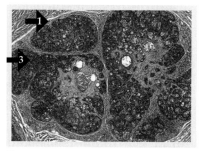

SEBACEOMA

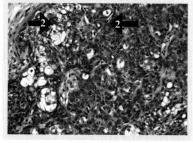

SEBACEOMA

HISTOLOGICAL DIFFERENTIAL

1. Sebaceous adenoma:
- More superficial than sebaceoma
- Seboblasts are localized at the periphery while mature sebocytes are present in the central part of the neoplasm and are the predominant cell
- Mitotic figures can be found in seboblasts but are not conspicuous
2. Sebaceous carcinoma:
- Usually large, asymmetric, poorly circumscribed
- Abundant necrosis (necrosis en masse)
- Nuclear atypia often striking
- Numerous and sometimes abnormal mitotic figures

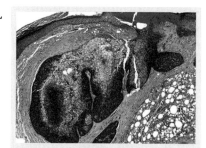

SEBACEOUS ADENOMA

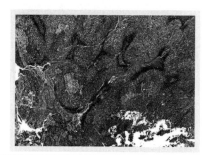

SEBACEOUS CARCINOMA

IMPORTANT THINGS TO KNOW

- There are scattered mitoses, but the tumor lacks prominent atypia
- Histopathologists should alert clinicians to the utility of having a patient with sebaceoma investigated for other cutaneous signs and internal evidence of Muir-Torre syndrome
- Muir-Torre syndrome is an inherited autosomal dominant germline mutation in one of the DNA mismatch repair (MMR) genes, most commonly *hMSH*

Sebaceous adenoma

Introduction

Sebaceous adenoma (SA) is a benign cutaneous neoplasm of the adnexa with sebaceous differentiation. A spectrum of morphologic features and varying degrees of differentiation can occur within one neoplasm.

Histological features

1. Multiple well-defined enlarged sebaceous lobules
2. Frequent attachment to epidermis with epidermal thinning
3. Small, undifferentiated, germinative basaloid cells at the periphery
4. Transitional cells and mature sebocytes in the center of the neoplasm
5. Varying ratio of basaloid and transitional cells to sebocytes, traditionally more than 50% are sebocytes
6. Lobules may contain duct-like structures

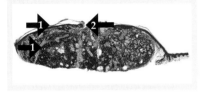
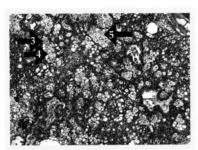

SEBACEOUS ADENOMA

Histological differential

1. Sebaceous hyperplasia:
- Has only one or two cell layers of germinative epithelium
- Relatively normal and uniform sebaceous lobules
2. Sebaceoma:
- More than 50% of cells are small germinative basaloid cells

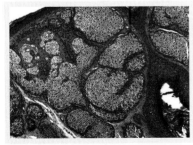

SEBACEOUS HYPERPLASIA

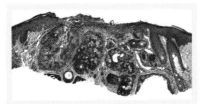

SEBACEOMA

Important things to know

- Histopathologists should alert clinicians to the utility of having a patient with sebaceous adenoma outside the face investigated for other cutaneous signs and internal evidence of Muir-Torre syndrome

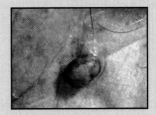

Epidemiology

- The exact incidence is unknown with no particular geographical location showing higher incidence rates
- No reported predisposition for any particular race
- Men and women are equally affected
- Most common on the face or scalp of middle-aged and older individuals (i.e. 50 years or greater)
- The mean age of onset is 60 years

Pathophysiology

- All sebaceous glands in the body have the potential to develop into sebaceous neoplasms. SAs are cutaneous adnexal tumors that show varying degrees of sebaceous differentiation

Clinical features

- Often a solitary yellow nodule found on the head, neck, and especially face of patients 50 years or older
- Gradual onset of small (<0.5 cm up to 5 cm plus), smooth, yellow papule/nodule, with possible polypoid appearance or central umbilication
- Occasionally, tumors may be seen at other sites, including the trunk and the legs
- Can be associated with Muir-Torre syndrome (characterized also by multiple sebaceous keratoacanthomas and visceral carcinomas, especially colonic adenocarcinoma)

Special studies

- No histologic features of SA could reliably pinpoint the association of Muir-Torre syndrome, but loss of nuclear staining for MLH-1 or MSH-2 suggests microsatellite instability and the syndrome

Clinical variants

- None

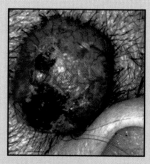

EPIDEMIOLOGY

- Unknown etiology
- Risk factors
  - o Older age
  - o Female
  - o Higher incidence in Caucasian, Asian, and Indians
  - o Irradiation
  - o Pre-existing sebaceous lesions
  - o Muir-Torre syndrome
  - o Immunosuppression

PATHOPHYSIOLOGY

- May originated from cells within sebaceous glands

CLINICAL FEATURES

- Most commonly presents as a painless, erythematous nodule or plaque that may be ulcerated or crusted, occasionally may display a yellowish coloration
- Early ocular lesions are very commonly misdiagnosed as blepharitis, chalazion or ocular rosacea
- About 75% occur in the periocular region but also occur elsewhere including head and neck and less commonly on the trunk

SPECIAL STUDIES

- EMA (epithelial membrane antigen) and adipophilin immunoperoxidase staining can be used to confirm sebaceous differentiation

CLINICAL VARIANTS

- None

SEBACEOUS CARCINOMA

INTRODUCTION

Sebaceous carcinoma is an aggressive, rare adnexal tumor characterized its tendency for local recurrence and metastasis. They usually manifest as a nodule but may have other clinical presentations, which may result in a delayed diagnosis.

HISTOLOGICAL FEATURES

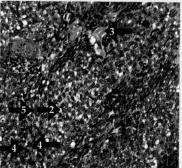

1. Irregular lobules or sheets of cells separated by a fibrovascular stroma
2. Variable sebaceous differentiation in the form of cells with vacuolated bubbly cytoplasm and scalloped nuclei
3. Necrosis which may be massive (necrosis en masse)
4. Neoplastic cells show marked nuclear pleomorphism and numerous mitotic figures, many of the atypical are identified
5. Smaller basaloid cells and squamous differentiation may be present

Other features:
- Pagetoid spread to the epidermis is seen in numerous cases

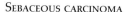

SEBACEOUS CARCINOMA

HISTOLOGICAL DIFFERENTIAL

1. Basal cell carcinoma:
- Smaller cells with more basophilic nuclei and smaller cytoplasm which is not vacuolated
- Less atypia
- Cells are more uniform
2. Sebaceoma:
- Circumscribed
- Symmetrical
- Higher percentage of differentiated to undifferentiated cells
- Less nuclear atypia and mitosis

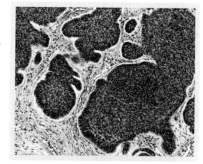

BASAL CELL CARCINOMA

IMPORTANT THINGS TO KNOW

- May be associated with the Muir-Torre syndrome
- Due to the pagetoid pattern, sebaceous carcinoma can be confused with pagetoid Bowen's disease and melanoma
- Sometimes the cells extend deeply and can involve the subcutaneous tissue and even the underlying muscle

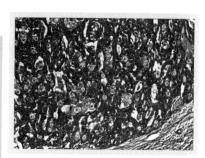

SEBACEOMA

APOCRINE ADENOMA

INTRODUCTION

Apocrine adenoma is a benign neoplasm which clinically presents as a smooth nonspecific nodules or papules and histologically as apocrine epithelium in either tubular or papillary patterns.

HISTOLOGICAL FEATURES

1. Circumscribed dermal tumor composed of lobules or tubules lined by apocrine epithelium
2. The neoplastic cells show an eosinophilic cytoplasm and areas of decapitation and secretion
3. Papillary projections without stroma into tubule's lumina

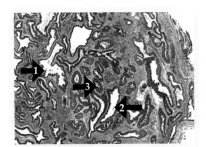

APOCRINE ADENOMA

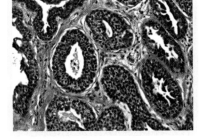

APOCRINE ADENOMA

HISTOLOGICAL DIFFERENTIAL

1. Hidradenoma papilliferum:
- Well-defined dermal nodular configuration
- An almost exclusive localization to the vulvar and perineal areas
- A predominance in women
2. Syringocystadenoma papilliferum:
- Prominent cystic invagination lined by squamoid and apocrine epithelium
- Prominent plasmacellular infiltrates in the stroma
- Localization to the head and neck area
- Frequent association with nevus sebaceus

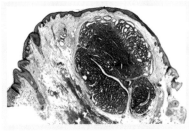
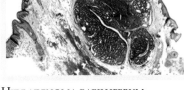

HIDRADENOMA PAPILLIFERUM

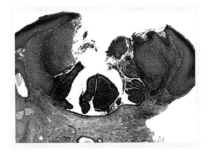

SYRINGOCYSTADENOMA PAPILLIFERUM

IMPORTANT THINGS TO KNOW

- Apocrine adenoma are always benign and excision is curative

EPIDEMIOLOGY

- Rare

PATHOPHYSIOLOGY

- Benign neoplasm arising from apocrine glands
- Unknown etiology

CLINICAL FEATURES

- Typically smooth nodule or papule
- Found on cheek, axillae, breast, genital, and perianal region or in association with an organoid nevus
- Biopsy required for diagnosis

SPECIAL STUDIES

- Immunoperoxidase staining for myoepithelial cells (S-100 and actin) helps to distinguish from adenocarcinoma

CLINICAL VARIANTS

- None

EPIDEMIOLOGY

- Rare
- Predominately affects children

PATHOPHYSIOLOGY

- Benign neoplasm arising from apocrine glands or pluripotential appendageal cells
- Unknown etiology

CLINICAL FEATURES

- 1–3 cm diameter
- Crusted, red warty plaque or nodule
- Usually found on head and neck though other locations are reported
- May ooze malodorous serosanguinous fluid
- Commonly found in conjunction with nevus sebaceous of Jadassohn (up to one-third of cases)

SPECIAL STUDIES

- CEA+
- GCDFP-15+
- CK7+

SYRINGOCYSTADENOMA PAPILLIFERUM

INTRODUCTION

Syringocystadenoma papilliferum is a benign apocrine neoplasm. These neoplasms present clinically as crusting and often oozing papules or plaques most commonly located on the head and neck. Histologically they are characterized by wide papillary fronds, which extend above the surface of the epidermis. The epithelium consists of oval to cuboidal cells with areas of decapitation and secretion.

HISTOLOGICAL FEATURES

1. Invaginating cystic spaces open to skin surface
2. Wide papillary fronds surfacing into epidermis
3. Frond bilayer consisting of basal cuboidal cells and apical columnar cells
4. Dense core of lymphocytes and plasma cells within stroma
5. Decapitation and secretion

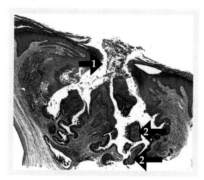
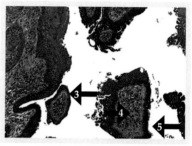

SYRINGOCYSTADENOMA PAPILLIFERUM

HISTOLOGICAL DIFFERENTIAL

1. Hidradenoma papilliferum:
- Usually less than 1 cm in diameter
- Most commonly found on vulva
- Well-demarcated nodular appearance in the dermis, usually without epidermal connection
- Less plasma cells in fibrous papillary cores
2. Nipple adenoma:
- Endophytic lesion, often open toward the epidermal surface
- Wedge-shaped and consists of tubular elements covered by a double row of epithelial cells
- Tubules are separated from one another by fibrous septa

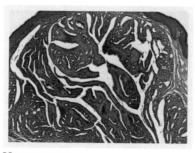
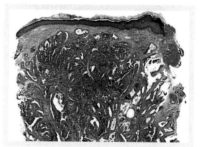

HIDRADENOMA PAPILLIFERUM   NIPPLE ADENOMA

IMPORTANT THINGS TO KNOW

- Rarely evolves into a carcinoma

CLINICAL VARIANTS

- None

Hidradenoma

Introduction

Hidradenoma is a form of benign adnexal neoplasm that is a close relative of poroma. It is usually characterized by cells with ample cytoplasm, and does not commonly have a broad-based connection to the epidermis. Hidradenomas can be either apocrine or eccrine lineage. The vast majority of hidradenomas are believed to be of apocrine lineage.

Histological features

1. Sharply circumscribed, non-encapsulated dermal tumor
2. Duct-like structures
3. Collections of cells with ample cytoplasm but uniform nuclei (larger than the nuclei of poroma)
4. Sclerotic stroma that may contain ectatic vessels
5. Cystic spaces may be present

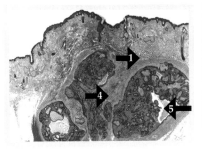 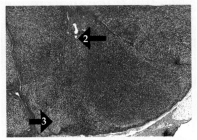 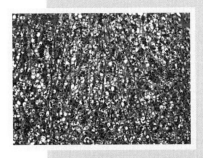

HIDRADENOMA

Histological differential

1. Poroma:
* Granulation tissue-like quality stroma
* Two populations of cells, poroid and cuticular
2. Metastatic renal cell carcinoma:
* Cells with ample eosinophilic cytoplasm
* Numerous blood vessels

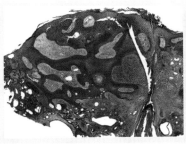 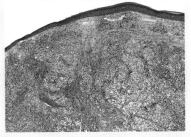

POROMA   METASTATIC RENAL CELL CARCINOMA

Important Things To Know

* Hybrid lesions with features of both hidradenoma and poroma can be encountered, and the intermediate term poroid hidradenoma has been applied in this setting

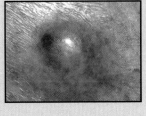

Epidemiology

* Any age
* More prominent in women than men

Pathophysiology

* Benign tumor with either apocrine or eccrine differentiation

Clinical features

* Solitary dermal or subcutaneous nodule
* Often skin-colored or blue-gray
* Sometimes, appears as a cystic lesion and produce serous drainage
* No anatomical preference

Special studies

* None

Clinical Variants

* None

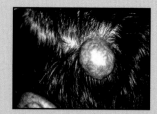

EPIDEMIOLOGY

- It may develop at any age but are most commonly in young adults, age 20–40 years
- More common in women

PATHOPHYSIOLOGY

- Familial cylindromatosis is inherited in an autosomal dominant fashion, and the responsible gene, *CYLD*, is located on chromosome 16q12-13

CLINICAL FEATURES

- Cylindroma is a firm or hard raised nodule, pink or bluish red in color, dome-shaped
- Most of the time they are solitary lesions that commonly involve the head and neck, especially the scalp
- However, multiple lesions can be also seen (turban tumor) cover the entire scalp, but they can also involve the face and upper body
- They are generally benign, but occasionally may show local invasion and malignant degeneration

SPECIAL STUDIES

- Immunohistochemical analysis: CK7, CK8, CK18, CEA are positive

CLINICAL VARIANTS

- Solitary
- Multiple sporadic
- Multiple as part of Brooke-Spiegler syndrome

CYLINDROMA

INTRODUCTION

A benign adnexal neoplasm, with a characteristic histology that usually manifests as nodules on the scalp.

HISTOLOGICAL FEATURES

1'. Dermal tumor without attachment to the epidermis
1. Basaloid cell islands in a jigsaw puzzle pattern
2. Two cellular population; outer layer composed of small, round cells with scant cytoplasm; inner layer composed of larger cells with more cytoplasm
3. Islands surrounded by sclerotic material and contain sweat ducts

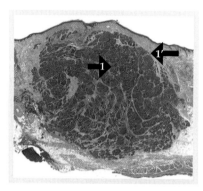 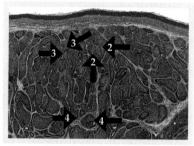

CYLINDROMA

HISTOLOGICAL DIFFERENTIAL

1. Spiradenoma:
- Prominent presence of lymphocytes
2. Basal cell carcinoma:
- Peripheral palisading
- Cleft between tumor and stroma
- Mucinous stroma
- Necrosis
- Mitoses

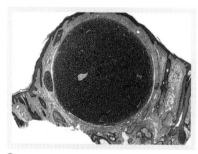 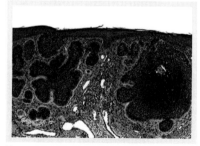

SPIRADENOMA   BASAL CELL CARCINOMA

IMPORTANT THINGS TO KNOW

- There are strong histochemical similarities between cylindromas and spiradenomas, and they may coexist in the same individual
- Cylindromas show an association with eccrine spiradenoma and trichoepitheliomas in Brooke syndrome

Apocrine hidrocystoma

Introduction

Apocrine hidrocystoma (AH) typically presents as translucent, skin-colored to bluish cysts on the face and histologically as unilocular or multilocular cysts lined by epithelial cells that demonstrate apocrine decapitation.

Histological features

1. Dermal cysts lined by two layers of epithelial cells
2. Outer layer of myoepithelial cells and inner layer of columnar with decapitation secretion

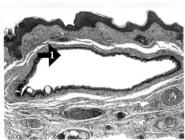
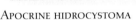

APOCRINE HIDROCYSTOMA

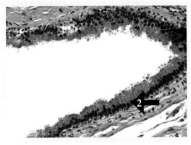

APOCRINE HIDROCYSTOMA

Histological differential

1. Epidermal inclusion cyst:
- Cystic cavity filled with laminated keratin
- Cyst lined by stratified squamous epithelium

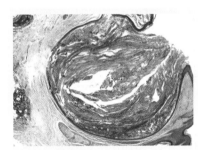

EPIDERMAL INCLUSION CYST

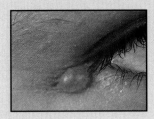

Epidemiology

- Occurs most commonly in middle-aged or elderly individuals

Pathophysiology

- It arises from the apocrine secretory coil

Clinical features

- Translucent, skin-colored to bluish cyst
- 3–15 mm diameter
- Typically found on face, neck, and periorbital region
- Usually solitary lesion
- Unusual in children

Special studies

- AH is S-100 negative, PAS positive; eccrine hidrocystomas are typically S-100 positive and PAS negative
- AH expresses human milk-fat globulin antigen while eccrine hidrocystomas do not

Important things to know

- May be associated with Schopf-Schulz-Passarge and Goltz syndrome

Clinical variants

- None

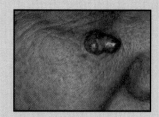

EPIDEMIOLOGY

- Rare
- More common in men

PATHOPHYSIOLOGY

- They are acquired hamartoma with folliculosebaceous-apocrine or eccrine differentiation

CLINICAL FEATURES

- Solitary, slow-growing nodule that are often misconstrued as cyst
- Commonly found in head and neck but may also develop in the trunk or in axillary or genital skin

SPECIAL STUDIES

- CEA

MIXED TUMOR

INTRODUCTION

Historically, mixed tumors of the skin, also known as chondroid syringoma, included both eccrine and apocrine variants. They are distinct benign adnexal neoplasms of the skin.

HISTOLOGICAL FEATURES

1. Well-circumscribed dermal or subcutaneous lobular tumor
2. Epithelial component: heterogeneous eccrine, apocrine, sebaceous, pilar, simple glandular, or squamous differentiation
3. Stromal component: variable chondroid, mucinous, hyalinized, or osteoid matrix

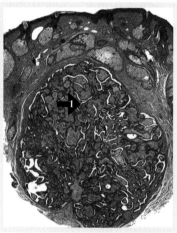
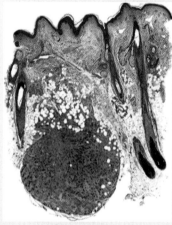

MIXED TUMOR APOCRINE TYPE   MIXED TUMOR ECCRINE TYPE

HISTOLOGICAL DIFFERENTIAL

1. Cutaneous chondroma:
- Absence of tubular structures
- Found in distal extremities (mixed tumors are more common in the head and neck)
- Prominent calcification

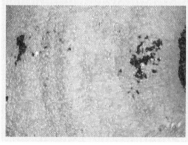

CHONDROMA

IMPORTANT THINGS TO KNOW

- Mixed tumor is benign and most lesions are treated by simple enucleation. In contrast to mixed tumors of salivary origin, there is no need for excision with wide margins.

CLINICAL VARIANTS

- None

SPIRADENOMA

INTRODUCTION

A spiradenoma is a benign adnexal tumor with areas of eccrine or apocrine origin. Usually lesions appear as solitary, slow-growing, tender or painful, reddish-brown or bluish intradermal nodule measuring 1–2 cm in diameter.

HISTOLOGICAL FEATURES

1. Sharply demarcated basophilic dermal nodule (blue balls in dermis)
2. No epidermal connection
3. Vascular stroma
4. A heavy diffuse lymphocytic infiltrate

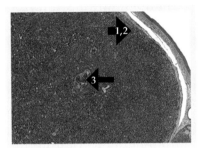 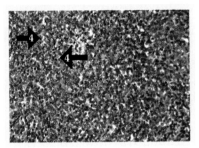

SPIRADENOMA   SPIRADENOMA

HISTOLOGICAL DIFFERENTIAL

1. Cylindroma:
   - Jigsaw puzzle
   - No lymphocytes
2. Basal cell carcinoma:
   - Originates from the epidermis, demonstrates peripheral palisading
   - Separation artifact (mucinous stroma)

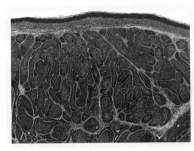 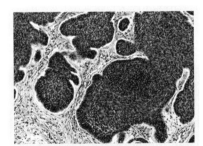

CYLINDROMA   BASAL CELL CARCINOMA

IMPORTANT THINGS TO KNOW

- Rarely, malignant progression may occur after benign lesions have been present for several months or several years
- Spiradenomas may be seen in Brooke-Spiegler syndrome
- An autosomal dominant condition associated with spiradenomas, multiple cylindromas and trichoepitheliomas/trichoblastomas

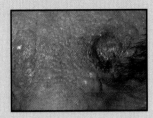

EPIDEMIOLOGY

- Mostly arises in young adults

PATHOPHYSIOLOGY

- It has either eccrine or apocrine differentiation

CLINICAL FEATURES

- Presents usually as a solitary dermal or subcutaneous papule or nodule, 1–2 cm in diameter, in a variety of hair bearing locations
- Nodules are usually tender and maybe painful
- Color may be reddish-brown or bluish
- Can simulate a vascular lesion
- Diagnosis may not be clear by clinical examination and a biopsy is usually warranted

SPECIAL STUDIES

- CEA may be positive

CLINICAL VARIANTS

- Solitary
- Multiple

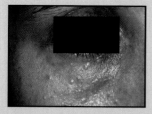

EPIDEMIOLOGY

- Syringomas often appear during the third and fourth decades of life, although, they are by no means limited to this time period and are commonly found in any age group at or after puberty
- They are twice as common in women
- More common in patients with Down syndrome

PATHOPHYSIOLOGY

- Syringomas arise from eccrine sweat glands

CLINICAL FEATURES

- Syringomas are small, skin-colored, often bilateral, firm papules. They are usually small and no larger than 1–2 mm in diameter
- Syringomas may occur at any site on the body but they mostly occur in the periorbital area, especially the eyelids
- They can also be found on the cheeks, axillae, vulva, penis and abdomen. The lesions on the vulva and penis are usually solitary
- Eruptive syringomas most commonly involve the trunk but may involve the extremities, including palms and soles

SPECIAL STUDIES

- None

CLINICAL VARIANTS

- Eruptive syringoma

SYRINGOMA

INTRODUCTION

Syringomas are small flesh-colored papules that are classically found on lower eyelids.

HISTOLOGICAL FEATURES

1. Well-defined superficial dermal tumor
2. Numerous small ducts embedded in sclerotic stroma
3. One or two layers of epithelial cells line the lumens of the ducts containing amorphous debris
4. Tadpole-shaped ducts

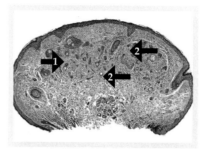
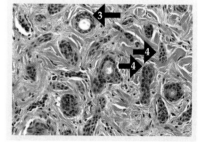

SYRINGOMA   SYRINGOMA

HISTOLOGICAL DIFFERENTIAL

1. Microcystic adnexal carcinoma:
- Large
- Deep infiltration of reticular dermis, subcutaneous fat, skeletal muscle, and cutaneous nerve
- Follicular differentiation
2. Desmoplastic trichoepithelioma:
- Fragments of keratin in the lumina
- Dystrophic calcification
- Rims of fibrous tissue around the neoplastic collections
- More frequent foreign body giant cell reaction to extruded keratin

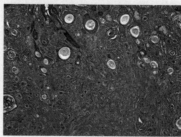
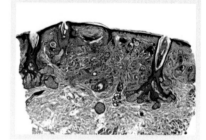

MICROCYSTIC ADNEXAL CARCINOMA   DESMOPLASTIC TRICHOEPITHELIOMA

IMPORTANT THINGS TO KNOW

- Rarely, syringoma will display cells clear, vacuolated cytoplasm. This is caused by accumulated glycogen and is known as clear cell syringoma and are associated with diabetes mellitus

POROMA

INTRODUCTION

Poroma is a benign adnexal neoplasm derived from acrosyringium. Histopathologically, poromas are traditionally subcategorized into three main variants based on their location in relation to the epidermis: hidroacanthoma simplex, poroma, and dermal duct tumor. The malignant counterpart of a poroma is known as porocarcinoma.

HISTOLOGICAL FEATURES

1. Well circumscribed
2. Connects with the epidermis
3. Mixture of small cuboidal cells with monomorphous ovoid nuclei (poroid cells) and larger cells with an eosinophilic cytoplasm (cuticular)
4. Ductal structures, consisting of tubules lined by a dense eosinophilic cuticle
5. Highly vascularized stroma, corresponding to a clinical picture similar to pyogenic granuloma

Main subtypes:
- Hidroacanthoma simplex represents a pattern of poroma in which tumor cells are confined to the epidermis
- Poroma involves both the epidermis and dermis. It consists of aggregates of uniform-looking basaloid cells radiating from the base of the epidermis into the dermis
- Dermal duct tumor is confined to the dermis. It consists of poroid cells forming several sharply circumscribed dermal nodules

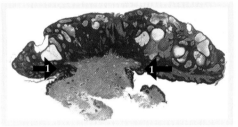 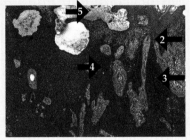

HISTOLOGICAL DIFFERENTIAL

1. Seborrheic keratosis:
- No ductal structures
- Horn pseudocysts
2. Basal cell carcinoma:
- Peripheral palisading
- Stromal retraction

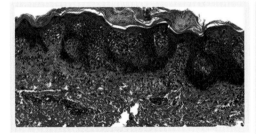

SEBORRHEIC KERATOSES

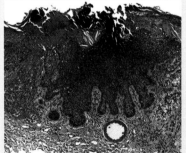

BASAL CELL CARCINOMA

IMPORTANT THINGS TO KNOW

- Poromas commonly display small collections of necrosis cells and the cause is unknown. Although necrosis en masse is suggestive of a malignancy (due to rapid growth beyond the capacity of perfusion), such occurrence in poromas is an exception

EPIDEMIOLOGY

- Onset of poromas is typically in adulthood but they can develop at any age
- No known gender or ethnic predisposition

PATHOPHYSIOLOGY

- Poromas are viewed as proliferations of the acrosyringium, which is the intraepidermal portion of the sweat duct

CLINICAL FEATURES

- Most commonly present as a solitary, slow-growing, papule/plaque or nodule on the soles or palms
- May be skin-colored, pigmented, or vascular in appearance, and sometimes exhibiting surface erosion or ulceration
- It may be itchy or painful

SPECIAL STUDIES

- None

CLINICAL VARIANTS

- None

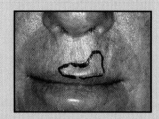

EPIDEMIOLOGY

- Female to male ratio of 3:2 with typical onset between 40–60 years of age
- Unknown etiology
- Risk factors unknown

PATHOPHYSIOLOGY

- ACC arises by neoplastic transformation of glandular epithelia stem cells. Initiating factor unknown

CLINICAL FEATURES

- Slow-growing mass invading dermis and subcutaneous tissue
- Typically found on scalp and chest area
- High incidence of local recurrence
- Perineural involvement and distant metastases in later stages of disease

SPECIAL STUDIES

- ACC is immunoreactive with epithelial membrane antigen (EMA) and carcinoembryonic antigen

ADENOID CYSTIC CARCINOMA

INTRODUCTION

Adenoid cystic carcinoma (ACC) is a rare malignant neoplasm associated with secretory glands throughout the body, including the salivary glands, respiratory tract, breast, skin, uterine cervix, thymus, and prostate gland. Commonly presented as a slow-growing mass, diagnosis is made histologically by biopsy and identification of their cribriform, tubular, or solid growth patterns.

HISTOLOGICAL FEATURES

1. Monomorphic basaloid cells with compact nuclei and a small amount of surrounding cytoplasm
2. Arranged in elongated nests, tubules and/or cords
3. Cribriform and tubular areas
4. Abundant basophilic mucin in cysts

Other features:
- Perineural infiltration

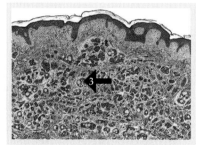
ADENOID CYSTIC CARCINOMA

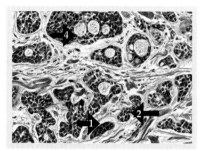
ADENOID CYSTIC CARCINOMA

HISTOLOGICAL DIFFERENTIAL

1. Adenoid basal cell carcinoma:
- Peripheral palisading
- Multilinear differentiation
- Stromal retraction

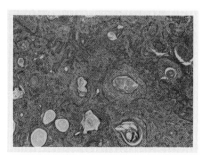
ADENOID BASAL CELL CARCINOMA

IMPORTANT THINGS TO KNOW

- Post-treatment, patients should be closely followed due to high recurrence rate

CLINICAL VARIANTS

- None

Microcystic adnexal carcinoma

Introduction

Microcystic adnexal carcinoma (MAC) is a rare cutaneous malignant tumor that is locally invasive and often presents with perineural invasion

Histological features

1. Biphasic pattern (sweat duct-like and pilar)
2. Tadpole-shaped ducts
3. Horn cysts
4. Sclerotic stroma
5. Deeply invasive, involves dermis and subcutis (bottom heavy)

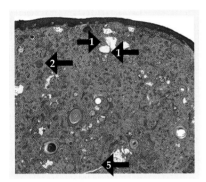 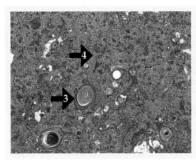

MICROCYSTIC ADNEXAL CARCINOMA

Histological differential

1. Syringoma:
- More superficial
- Small
- No perineural extension
- No lymphoid aggregation
2. Desmoplastic trichoepithelioma:
- More superficial
- No perineural extension
- Rare lymphoid aggregation

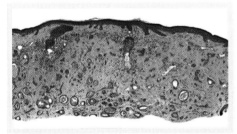 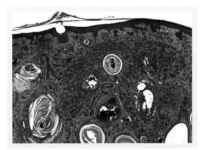

SYRINGOMA

DESMOPLASTIC TRICHOEPITHELIOMA

IMPORTANT THINGS TO KNOW

- MAC is a low-grade form of adnexal carcinoma
- Local recurrence common
- Metastasis rare
- Perineural invasion and lymphoid aggregates sometimes are seen in MAC

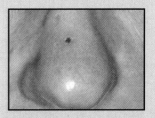

Epidemiology

- Typically seen in young or middle-aged adults
- More prominent in women than men
- Risk factors: UV light exposure

Pathophysiology

- It is a carcinoma that differentiates toward sweat glands and hair follicles

Clinical features

- Slow growing
- Indurated, firm plaque or nodule
- Yellow to flesh-colored
- Predilection for face, head, and neck (most commonly on the upper lip)
- Typically presents on the left side

Special studies

- CEA, EMA, CK7

Clinical variants

- None

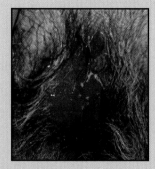

EPIDEMIOLOGY

- EMPD represents 1–2% of primary neoplasms of the vulva and anogenital region. Axillae, eyelids and external auditory canal rarely may be involved
- Women are commonly affected. Most patients are above the age of 60

PATHOPHYSIOLOGY

- It is thought to arise from pluripotential stem cells in the epidermis
- It can be associated with an underlying adenocarcinoma of skin appendages or Bartholin's glands
- EMPD needs to be distinguished from secondary pagetoid colonization of the epidermis by a noncutaneous carcinoma, mainly from the bladder or the bowel

CLINICAL FEATURES

- Well-demarcated erythematous scaly patches and plaques, which may be ulcerated
- Intractable pruritis is a common presenting symptom

SPECIAL STUDIES

- Immunohistochemical analysis: CK7+, CAM5.2+, EMA+, pCEA+, GCDFP15+, HER2+, stains for mucin are positive in 70% of the cases

CLINICAL VARIANTS

- None

EXTRAMAMMARY PAGET'S DISEASE

INTRODUCTION

Extramammary Paget's disease (EMPD) is an uncommon intraepithelial adenocarcinoma, which primarily affects the apocrine-bearing skin.

HISTOLOGICAL FEATURES

1. Neoplastic cells with large nuclei and abundant amphophilic cytoplasm
2. Single cells or clusters more numerous in basal layer
3. Glandular structures commonly seen

Other features:
- Tumor cells with propensity to track along skin appendages

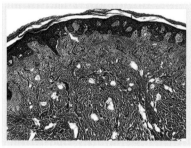

EXTRAMAMMARY PAGET'S DISEASE

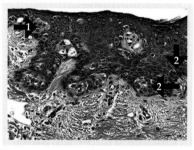

EXTRAMAMMARY PAGET'S DISEASE

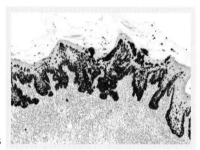

CK7 STAINING

HISTOLOGICAL DIFFERENTIAL

1. Pagetoid squamous cell carcinoma in situ:
- CK5/6+, P63+, CK7–, CEA–, GCDFP15–
2. Melanoma in situ:
- S-100+, HMB-45+, CK7–, CEA–, GCDFP15–

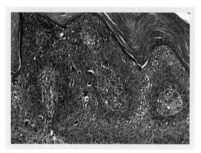

PAGETOID SQUAMOUS CELL CARCINOMA IN SITU

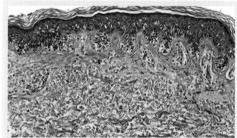

MELANOMA IN SITU

IMPORTANT THINGS TO KNOW

- Paget cells can contain cytoplasmic melanin pigment, a feature that should not imply melanocytic differentiation

Hidradenocarcinoma

Introduction

Hidradenocarcinoma is a rare malignant carcinoma often appearing on the face and extremities, and sometimes trunk. Most cases develop de novo and rarely in association with an existent hidradenoma. Clinically, it is very hard to diagnose due to the variations of its presentation.

Histological features

1. Sheets of cells with glycogen-containing pale cytoplasm and distinct cell membranes
2. Cytoplasmic vacuoles
3. Focal necrosis

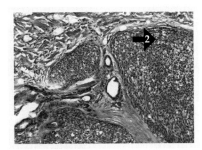

HIDRADENOCARCINOMA

Histological differential

1. Porocarcinoma:
- Lack of clear cell change
2. Sebaceous carcinoma:
- Sebaceous differentiation (vacuolated cells)

SEBACEOUS CARCINOMA

POROCARCINOMA

IMPORTANT THINGS TO KNOW

- Aggressive course, with distant metastasis to lymph nodes, bones, and lungs
- Wide local excision with 2 cm margins is the treatment of choice

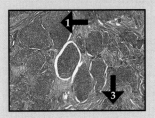

EPIDEMIOLOGY

- Common in middle-aged to elderly

PATHOPHYSIOLOGY

- Most tumors have apocrine differentiation

CLINICAL FEATURES

- Usually presents as an ulcerated reddish nodule in elderly

SPECIAL STUDIES

- Cam5.2+, EMA decorate the luminal border of ductal structures

CLINICAL VARIANTS

- None

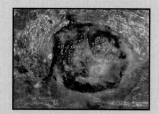

EPIDEMIOLOGY

- Porocarcinomas represent 0.005–0.01% of all malignant cutaneous tumors
- It is primarily a tumor of elderly adults, 50–80 years of age, although it has been reported in young adults
- There is no predilection for either gender

PATHOPHYSIOLOGY

- The etiology of theses tumors remains unknown, they can arise de novo or in a pre-existing benign poroma

CLINICAL FEATURES

- The lesions present as nodules or infiltrated plaques with or without verrucous, ulcerative or polypoid characteristics
- Most frequent sites of involvement are the lower extremities followed by the trunk and head
- Tumors vary in size from 1 cm to 10 cm. A long standing history is often encountered
- The incidence of lymph nodes metastasis and distant metastasis are 20% and 11%, respectively. Recurrence rate after excisions 20%

SPECIAL STUDIES

- Immunohistochemical analysis: Ductal differentiation can be highlighted by EMA and CEA

CLINICAL VARIANTS

- None

POROCARCINOMA

INTRODUCTION

Porocarcinoma is a rare aggressive malignant adnexal neoplasm of sweat gland duct.

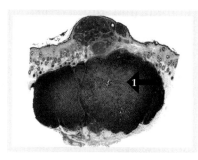
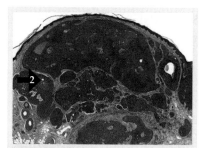

HISTOLOGICAL FEATURES

1. Cords and lobules of invasive pleomorphic basaloid cells
2. Ducts lined by cuboidal epithelial cells and eosinophilic luminal cuticle
3. Frequent mitoses and sometimes necrosis
4. Squamous differentiation and clear cell changes

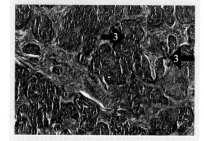

POROCARCINOMA

HISTOLOGICAL DIFFERENTIAL

1. Squamous cell carcinoma:
- No evidence of ductal differentiation
- No poroid cells
2. Poroma:
- Well circumscribed and symmetrical
- No atypia

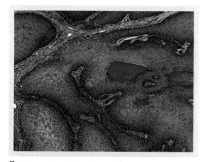

SQUAMOUS CELL CARCINOMA

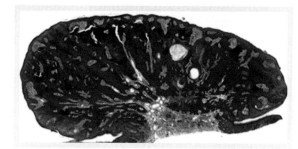

POROMA

IMPORTANT THINGS TO KNOW

- Ducts lined by cuboidal cells and eosinophilic cuticle help to differentiate porocarcinoma from other malignant tumors

TUMORS OF FIBROUS TISSUE

BENIGN TUMORS • NODULAR FASCIITIS

INTRODUCTION

Nodular fasciitis is a benign reactive proliferation of fibroblast-like cells that appears as a well-circumscribed, subcutaneous, fascial or intramuscular nodule.

HISTOLOGICAL FEATURES

1. Spindle-shaped to plump fibroblasts and myofibroblasts in a haphazard arrangement ("tissue culture appearance") embedded in a mucinous stroma
2. Cells with prominent oval nuclei and fine chromatin pattern
3. Lymphocytes and extravasated red cells are also seen

Other features:
- Typical mitoses are common
- Some cells may have a ganglion like appearance
- Capillaries with plump endothelial cells
- Ossifying fasciitis shows areas with osteoid metaplasia

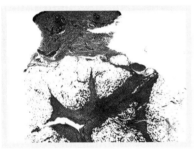

NODULAR FASCIITIS

NODULAR FASCIITIS

HISTOLOGICAL DIFFERENTIAL

1. Fibrosarcoma:
- Proliferation of atypical fibroblasts arranged in a herringbone pattern. No mucinous stroma
2. Pleomorphic sarcoma (malignant fibrous histiocytoma):
- Neoplasms composed of pleomorphic cells of different sizes and shapes

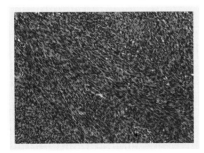

FIBROSARCOMA

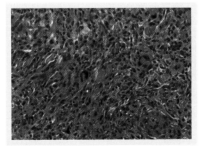

MALIGNANT FIBROUS HISTIOCYTOMA

IMPORTANT THINGS TO KNOW

- Nodular fasciitis can become very large and recur, especially in areas like the head and neck
- Cells of nodular fasciitis produce tyrosine kinase, transforming growth factor β, interferon, and tumor necrosis factor

EPIDEMIOLOGY

- Common among soft tissue mass lesions
- Affects all age groups but more often young adults
- Intravascular fasciitis and cranial fasciitis are rare
- Intravascular fasciitis is found mostly in persons under 30 years of age
- Cranial fasciitis develops predominantly in infants under 2 years of age
- No sex predilection but cranial fasciitis is more frequent in boys

PATHOPHYSIOLOGY

- Some patients with nodular fasciitis report trauma to the site of the lesion, but the majority do not
- Birth trauma may be a factor in the genesis of cranial fasciitis

CLINICAL FEATURES

- Most commonly affects young to middle-aged adults in the upper extremities
- Cranial fasciitis is a variant found in children; arises in deep tissues of the scalp and involves cranium
- Lesions may grow quickly to >5 cm in diameter
- Self-limited process

SPECIAL STUDIES

- Immunoperoxidase studies: cells are positive for smooth muscle actin, muscle-specific actin, vimentin, KP-1; negative for desmin and S-100 protein
- Ganglion cells are only positive for vimentin

CLINICAL VARIANTS

- Florid reactive periostitis or fibro-osseous pseudotumor of the digits

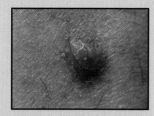

EPIDEMIOLOGY

- Dermatofibroma is a very common lesion and may develop at any age
- There is a predilection for the extremities, particularly the lower of young adults
- There is a female predominance

PATHOPHYSIOLOGY

- It is controversial whether it is an inflammatory or neoplastic process
- Dermatofibroma has been reported following local injuries such as trauma, insect bites, or folliculitis, suggesting an inflammatory etiology
- By contrast, some examples have been reported to be clonal, supportive of a neoplastic etiology

CLINICAL FEATURES

- Dermatofibromas are round or ovoid, firm dermal nodules
- Usually less than 1 cm in diameter
- It preferentially develops on the lower limbs
- Usually a dusky brown color but aneurysmal variants may be red, and tumors with abundant lipid can be cream/yellow
- Most often solitary

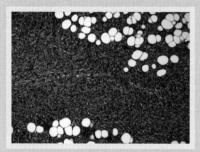 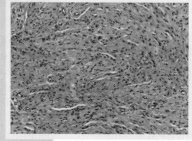

DERMATOFIBROSARCOMA PROTUBERANS   NEUROFIBROMA

SPECIAL STUDIES

- Immunohistochemistry: cells are usually positive for factor XIIIa

CLINICAL VARIANTS

- None

DERMATOFIBROMA

INTRODUCTION

Dermatofibromas (DF), also known as benign fibrous histiocytomas, are common cutaneous nodules of unknown etiology. There are a number of histologic subtypes. Tumors that grow deeply into the fat underlying the skin do have the potential for aggressive growth and local recurrence.

HISTOLOGICAL FEATURES

1. Well-circumscribed neoplasm that usually spares the papillary dermis and subcutaneous tissue and is perpendicular to the epidermis
2. Epidermal hyperplasia with flattened "tabled rete ridges" and hyperpigmentation of the basal layer
3. Follicular (simulating a basal cell carcinoma) and sebaceous induction
4. Fibroblast of different size and shape and multinucleated histiocytes in many cases
5. Prominent kelloidal collagen at the periphery

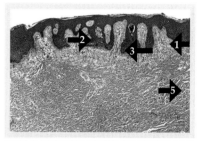

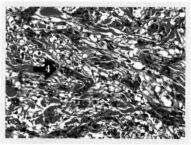

DERMATOFIBROMA

Other features:
- Hemosiderin in the aneurysmal variant
- Histological variants: aneurysmal/hemosiderotic dermatofibroma, cellular dermatofibroma, deep fibrous histiocytoma, atypical fibrous histiocytoma/dermatofibroma with monster cells and sclerotic DF

HISTOLOGICAL DIFFERENTIAL

1. Dermatofibrosarcoma protuberans:
- Large and poorly circumscribed, parallel to the epidermis
- Bundles of collagen arranged in a storiform pattern and trapping subcutaneous fat
- Cells with wavy nuclei in association with delicate fibrillary bundles
  - CD34 positive
2. Neurofibroma:
  - Spindle cells with wavy nuclei admixed with a variable number of mast cells
  - Mucinous stroma
  - No keloidal collagen
  - Immunoreactive for S-100 protein and neurofilament

IMPORTANT THINGS TO KNOW

- They often show a characteristic central white, scar-like patch on dermatoscopic examination, and a delicate pigment network at the periphery
- Many lesions demonstrate a "dimple sign," where the central portion puckers as the lesion is compressed on the sides. They generally do not change in size
- Cellular DF may be CD34 positive

Superficial Fibromatosis

Introduction

Fibromatosis have been defined as a "group of non-metastasizing fibrous tumors which tend to be locally aggressive and recur after surgical excision". The "fibromatosis" include entities such as palmar and plantar fibromatosis, and Peyronie's disease of the penis, and knuckle pads.

Histological features

1. Hypercellular lesions composed of fusiform fibroblasts with vesiculous nuclei
2. Stroma with moderate amount of collagen

Other features:
• In early stages mitotic figures can be seen

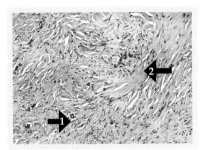

FIBROMATOSIS

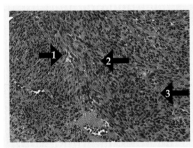

FIBROMATOSIS

Histological differential

1. Dermatofibrosarcoma protuberans:
• Infiltrative neoplasms with monotonous cells in a storiform pattern extending into the subcutaneous fat and producing a honeycomb appearance
2. Leiomyomas:
• Centered in reticular dermis but may extend into subcutaneous fat
• Fascicles of smooth muscle and collagen

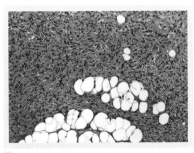

DERMATOFIBROSARCOMA PROTUBERANS

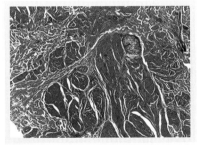

LEIOMYOMA

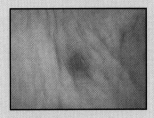

Epidemiology

• May occur in childhood or be acquired in adulthood
• Some patients may have more than one of fibromatosis at the same time

Pathophysiology

• Proliferation of well-differentiated fibroblasts, an infiltrative growth pattern, and aggressive clinical behavior with frequent local recurrence

Clinical features

• Plantar fibromatosis: young to middle-aged adults, thick sole may interfere with walking
• Palmar fibromatosis (Dupuytren's contracture): older males, often develops clinically chord-like bands on the palms with flexion contraction
• Penile fibromatosis (Peyronie's disease): middle-aged to older adult males slowly develop fibrous thickening of penis often with dorsal curvature of the penis with pain
• Knuckle pads affects dorsum of the hands at the interphalangeal joints affecting mostly young adults and middle-aged

Special studies

• Immunohistochemical studies demonstrate that the neoplastic cells are positive for vimentin, smooth muscle actin and some positivity for β-catenin

Important Things To Know

• Multiple fibromatoses are seen in Gardener's a syndrome
• Treatment is mainly surgical

Clinical Variants

• Plantar fibromatosis
• Palmar fibromatosis
• Knuckle pads
• Peyronie's disease

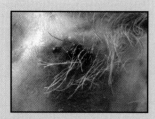

EPIDEMIOLOGY

- The incidence of this tumor is difficult to assess because it is mostly a diagnosis of exclusion
- It probably accounts for 1–3% of adult sarcomas
- Classical fibrosarcoma is most common in middle-aged and older adults
- Congenital or infantile fibrosarcoma is present at birth or develops within the first year of life
- The sex incidence is equal

PATHOPHYSIOLOGY

- Some arise in the field of previous therapeutic irradiation, and rarely in association with implanted foreign material
- Thermal burns, radiation therapy may lead to cutaneous fibrosarcomas
- Congenital-infantile fibrosarcoma presents with a translocation t(12;15)(p13;q25) leads to *ETV6–NTRK3* gene fusion

CLINICAL FEATURES

- Fibrosarcoma presents as a mass with or without pain
- In specific sites local symptoms relate to the effects of a mass
- Affects young to middle-aged adults
- Usually located in lower extremities, followed by the upper extremities, trunk, and then the head and neck region
- Hemorrhage and necrosis can be seen in high grade tumors

SPECIAL STUDIES

- Tumor cells express vimentin but not desmin, S-100 protein, or smooth muscle actin

CLINICAL VARIANTS

- Congenital or infantile fibrosarcoma

INTRODUCTION

A fibrosarcoma is a malignant tumor of fibroblasts with no other cellular differentiation. The greater the cellularity and the number of mitotic figures, the more aggressive the neoplasm. The most aggressive fibrosarcomas can metastasize, especially to the lungs via blood stream.

HISTOLOGICAL FEATURES

1. Interlacing fascicles of spindle cells in a "herringbone pattern"
2. Scant cytoplasm and elongated hyperchromatic nuclei
3. Meshwork of collagen and reticulin between cells

Other features:
- Mitotic figures
- Histologic variants: sclerosing epithelioid fibrosarcoma, fibrosarcoma with palisaded granuloma-like bodies (giant rosettes), and inflammatory fibrosarcoma

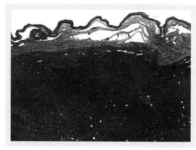

FIBROSARCOMA

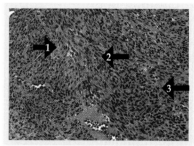

FIBROSARCOMA

HISTOLOGICAL DIFFERENTIAL

1. Malignant fibrous histiocytoma:
- Partial fibroblastic and histiocytic differentiation
- Collagen production
- Multinucleated cells usually present
2. Nodular fasciitis:
- Involves myofibroblasts as well as fibroblasts
- Common in the upper extremities
- May express KP-1

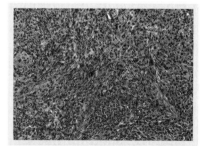

MALIGNANT FIBROUS HISTIOCYTOMA

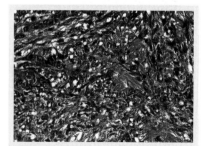

NODULAR FASCIITIS

IMPORTANT THINGS TO KNOW

- Congenital-infantile fibrosarcoma: less aggressive than adult-type. Histological appearance is similar
- Tumors with the histological features of adult fibrosarcoma may arise in dermatofibrosarcoma, solitary fibrous tumor and in well-differentiated liposarcoma, either in the primary or in recurrence, as a reflection of tumor dedifferentiation

Dermatofibrosarcoma Protuberans

Introduction

Dermatofibrosarcoma protuberans (DFSP) is a locally aggressive sarcoma of low-intermediate malignancy that favors young to middle-aged adults. Lesions that are present at birth or with an onset during childhood have been reported. DFSP occurs on the trunk in 50–60% of patients, the proximal extremities in 20–30%, and the head and neck in 10–15%. There is a predilection for the shoulder or pelvic region.

Histological features

1. Poorly circumscribed neoplasm which has a parallel orientation to the epidermis
2. Affects dermis and extends into the subcutaneous tissue
3. Has a characteristic honeycomb pattern with trapping of the subcutaneous tissue
4. The cells are fairly uniform

Other features:
- Mitotic figures are low-to-moderate (less than 5/10 HPF)
- Tumor cells tightly encase skin appendages without destroying them
- Some tumors have a prominent myxoid matrix
- In some tumors, multinucleated cells are seen (giant cell fibroblastoma)

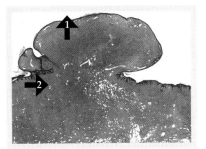 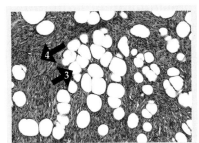

Dermatofibrosarcoma protuberans

Histological differential

1. Fibrosarcoma:
- Highly pleomorphic cells
- Herringbone pattern
2. Dermatofibroma (especially deep penetrating variants):
- Epidermal hyperplasia
- Extension into the subcutaneous tissue
- Keloidal collagen and multinucleated histiocytes
- Positive staining for factor XIIIa and negative staining for CD34 in most cases

Fibrosarcoma

Important Things To Know

- Treatment of choice: Mohs micrographic surgery
- Multiple local recurrences appear to lead to the evolution of a more aggressive tumors and the development of a metastatic disease

---

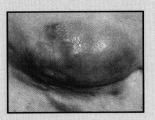

Epidemiology

- DFSP typically presents during early or middle adult life However, some tumors start during childhood and become only apparent during young adulthood
- Male predominance

Pathophysiology

- Unique cytogenetic abnormalities reciprocal t(17;22) translocations
- DFSP arises from the dermis and invades deeper subcutaneous tissue (fat, fascia, muscle, bone)
- The cellular origin of DFSP is uncertain
- A history of precedent trauma is present in 10–20% of all patients
- DFSP may also arise in surgical scars, burns and vaccination sites

Clinical features

- It presents as a slowly growing, asymptomatic, skin-colored, indurated plaque
- Violaceous to red–brown nodules measuring from one to several centimeters in diameter
- On palpation, the lesion is firm and attached to the subcutaneous tissue
- Accelerated growth during pregnancy
- Most common locations: trunk and proximal extremities

Special studies

- Immunostaining pattern of DFSP: CD34-positive, factor XIIIa-negative

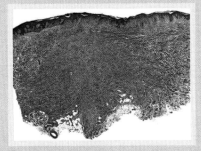

Dermatofibroma

Clinical Variants

- Bednar tumor
- Myxoid DFSP
- Giant cell fibroblastoma

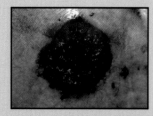

Epidemiology

- Predominance in elderly males
- A few in children with xeroderma pigmentosum
- A rare variant can develop in non-sun-damaged skin of the trunk or extremities in younger patients

Pathophysiology

- It has been regarded as a proliferative mesenchymal, possibly fibrohistiocytic, response to a variety of cutaneous injuries
- In older patients there is often a history of prolonged actinic exposure, but lesions may also develop at sites of irradiation and even trauma
- This tumor may also develop in renal transplant recipients
- A less aggressive behavior has been associated to the absence of *ras* oncogene mutations in AFX, whereas MFH has both H- and K-ras gene mutations
- Neoplasm that extend into the subcutaneous tissue have a higher incidence of recurrence
- Lesions may regress spontaneously or after incomplete removal

Clinical features

- It usually presents as a solitary rapidly growing nodule
- Gray to pink or red dome-shaped nodule that measures from 1–2 cm in diameter on the head or neck of the elderly
- Secondary changes include serosanguineous crusts and ulceration may occur

Special studies

- Both the spindle-shaped cells and the histiocyte-like cells react positively for vimentin
- The large histiocyte-like cells react positively for α1-antichymotrypsin, CD68, procollagen and CD10
- Negative for Pankeratin and S-100

Clinical Variants

- None

Atypical fibroxanthoma (superficial malignant fibrous histiocytoma)

Introduction

Atypical fibroxanthoma is a low-grade sarcoma that occurs in sun-damaged skin of the head and neck of elderly patients. Atypical fibroxanthoma is considered to be a superficial form of malignant fibrous histiocytoma.

Histological features

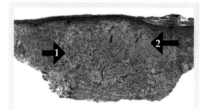

1. Poorly circumscribed neoplasm composed of pleomorphic cells, which affect the dermis and sometimes extend into the subcutaneous tissue
2. Solar elastosis
3. Atypical bizarre spindle-shaped cells and multinucleated cells

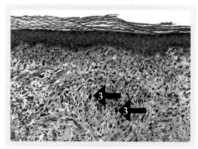

Other features:
- Often the epidermis is ulcerated
- Numerous mitotic figures
- Large atypical cells with abundant pale-staining vacuolated cytoplasm
- A rare variant with scattered osteoclast-like multinucleated giant cells has been reported

ATYPICAL FIBROXANTHOMA

Histological differential

1. Leiomyosarcoma:
- Nuclear atypia
- Mitotic activity of 1 or more per 50 HPF
- Necrosis
- Positive SMA
2. Desmoplastic melanoma:
- Focal lymphoid aggregate
- Positive S-100 and P75 but negative Melan-A and HMB-45

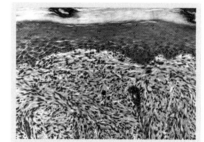

LEIOMYOSARCOMA

Important Things To Know

- Features that may portend a more aggressive behavior include vascular invasion (the most reliable feature), extension into deep tissues and tumor necrosis which is more prominent in MFH
- Atypical fibroxanthomas should be treated by wide local excision, Mohs technique may be of benefit in cases on the head and neck

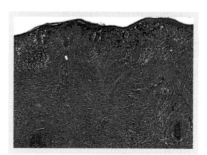

DESMOPLASTIC MELANOMA

TUMORS OF FAT

LIPOMA

INTRODUCTION

Lipoma is a benign tumor composed of mature adipocytes and is the most common soft tissue mesenchymal neoplasm in adults.

HISTOLOGICAL FEATURES

1. Lobules of mature adipocytes, surrounded by a delicate connective tissue
2. Cells are identical to the surrounding adipose tissue

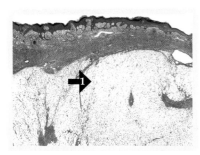

LIPOMA

HISTOLOGICAL DIFFERENTIAL

1. Angiolipoma:
- Prominent blood vessels
2. Spindle cell lipoma:
- Prominent spindle cells in mucinous stroma in adipose tissue

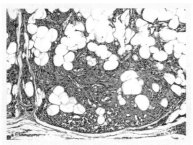

ANGIOLIPOMA

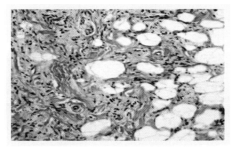

SPINDLE CELL LIPOMA

IMPORTANT THINGS TO KNOW

- The infiltrating intramuscular lipoma has a higher local recurrence rate, therefore total removal of the involved muscle or a compartmental resection has been suggested for these infiltrating tumors in order to minimize local recurrence

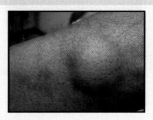

EPIDEMIOLOGY

- Most common between the ages of 40 and 60 years
- More frequent in obese individuals
- Rare in children
- Approximately 5% of patients have multiple lipomas

PATHOPHYSIOLOGY

- Unknown, however, lipomas are more common in obese individuals

CLINICAL FEATURES

- Lipomas are usually painless, except for larger ones that can elicit pain if they compress peripheral nerves
- Superficial lipomas are generally smaller (<5 cm) than the deep seated ones (>5 cm)
- Lipoma arborescens is a fatty infiltration of subsynovial connective tissue in a large joint, usually the knee. Affects older patients, usually male, associated with joint trauma, degenerative joint disease and chronic arthritis
- Conventional lipoma can arise within subcutaneous tissue (superficial lipoma) or within deep soft tissues (deep lipoma) or even on the surfaces of bone (parosteal lipoma)
- Deep-seated lipomas that arise within or between skeletal muscle fibers are called intramuscular or intermuscular lipomas, respectively

SPECIAL STUDIES

- Mature adipocytes stain for vimentin, S-100 protein and leptin
- Imaging studies show a homogeneous soft tissue mass that is isodense to the subcutaneous tissue and demonstrates fat saturation

CLINICAL VARIANTS

- Conventional lipoma
- Deep-seated lipoma

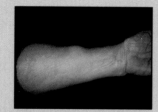

EPIDEMIOLOGY

- Angiolipomas comprise 10% of tumors of the fat
- Occur at young age group

PATHOPHYSIOLOGY

- Angiolipomas have normal karyotype, and for this reason they have been regarded as a hamartoma of blood vessels and fat, rather than a true tumor of fat
- A family history is found in about 10% of cases

CLINICAL FEATURES

- Painful lesions occur most commonly in the forearm or on the trunk
- Usually multiple

SPECIAL STUDIES

- None

CLINICAL VARIANTS

- None

ANGIOLIPOMA

INTRODUCTION

Angiolipomas are subcutaneous tumors of blood vessels and fat.

HISTOLOGICAL FEATURES

1. Thin fibrous capsule with incomplete fibrous septa
2. Variable proportion of mature adipose and blood vessels
3. Fibrin micro thrombi

Cellular angiolipoma:
- Vascular component comprises the bulk of the lesion

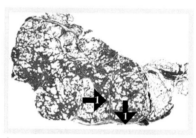

ANGIOLIPOMA

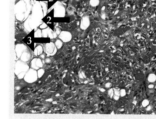

ANGIOLIPOMA

HISTOLOGICAL DIFFERENTIAL

1. Lipoma:
- No fibrin thrombi
2. Hemangioma:
- Capillaries radiate out from a central large vessel but in angiolipoma, capillaries are located peripherally

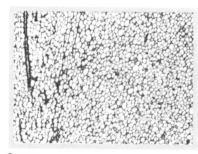

LIPOMA

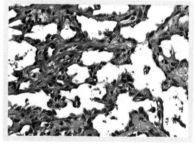

HEMANGIOMA

Nevus lipomatosus superficialis

Introduction

Nevus lipomatosus superficialis (NLS) is an uncommon form of connective tissue nevus, manifest principally by the deposition of fatty tissue in the dermis.

Histological features

1. Polypoid lesion made up of lobules of mature fat in variable quantities in superficial dermis
2. Increased number of small blood vessels around fatty lobules
3. Areas of loose fibrous tissue

Other features:
• Diminished elastic fibers and reduced numbers of epidermal appendages

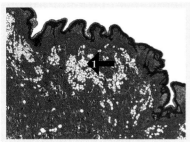
Nevus lipomatosus superficialis

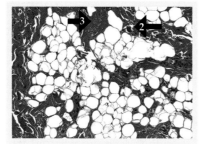
Nevus lipomatosus superficialis

Histological differential

1. Fibroepithelial polyp:
• Papillary, fibrovascular cores covered by squamous epithelium
• May have ischemic necrosis due to torsion

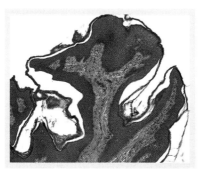
Skin tag

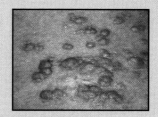

Epidemiology

• Typically, the lesions present in early childhood or adolescence
• Such lesions have been described as pedunculated lipofibroma
• In all types of nevus lipomatosus the sex incidence is equal

Pathophysiology

• The pathogenesis is unknown

Clinical features

• In classical form, it is characterized by multiple papular, polypoid, or plaque-like lesions, up to 2 cm in diameter, which almost always arise unilaterally on the posterior surfaces of the buttocks, upper thighs or lower back
• The papules or plaques, varying from skin-colored to yellow, are characteristically broad based and may show superficial comedone formation

Special studies

• None

Clinical Variants

• Solitary form NLS
• Extensive and diffuse NLS

Important Things To Know

• A solitary form, usually seen in adults, shows a predilection for the same sites or occurs elsewhere and is more likely to represent a variant of fibroepithelial polyp or skin tag

TUMORS OF SMOOTH MUSCLE

BENIGN NEOPLASMS • LEIOMYOMA

EPIDEMIOLOGY

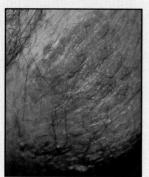

- Uncommon
- Females more often affected than males
- Congenital lesions are probably variants of smooth muscle hamartoma

PATHOPHYSIOLOGY

- Leiomyomas arise from smooth muscle cells
- Most patients with multiple leiomyomas have germline mutation of the fumarate hydratase gene

CLINICAL FEATURES

- Piloleiomyomas: Mostly seen in adults, solitary or multiple, painful, firm, reddish-brown papules or nodules. Usually 1–2 cm in diameter. Multiple nodules often seen as plaques, linear, grouped, or in a dermatomal pattern. Appear more often in lower extremities and trunk (especially shoulder)
- Genital leiomyomas: Often solitary, painless, well-circumscribed subcutaneous nodules. Usually <2 cm in diameter but may be as large as 15 cm in diameter. Appear on vulva, penis, scrotum, nipple and areola

LEIOMYOMA (SUPERFICIAL LEIOMYOMA/ LEIOMYOMA CUTIS/SUPERFICIAL BENIGN SMOOTH MUSCLE TUMOR)

INTRODUCTION

Leiomyomas are benign dermal tumors that are subclassified into three categories according to their location. Piloleiomyomas arise from the erector pili muscles; genital leiomyomas arise in the dartos, vulvar, or mammillary smooth muscles; and angioleiomyomas arise in the smooth muscle of blood vessel walls.

HISTOLOGICAL FEATURES

1. Neoplasm composed of uniform smooth muscle cells with eosinophilic cytoplasm, oval nuclei with blunt ends "cigar"-shaped

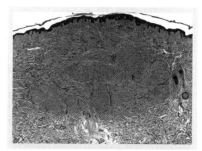

Piloleiomyomas
- Usually centered in reticular dermis but may extend into surrounding fat tissue, or subcutis
- Poorly circumscribed fascicles of smooth muscle and collagen (unencapsulated and infiltrative) often involving hair follicles and adnexal glands

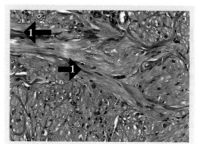

Genital leiomyomas
- Well circumscribed and centered in subcutaneous tissue
- Spindle-shaped or epithelioid cells, may have a pseudocapsule, focal calcifications, or stromal myxoid change. Few mitotic figures may be present

LEIOMYOMA

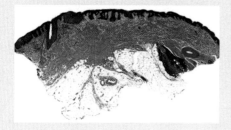

DERMATOFIBROMA

LEIOMYOSARCOMA

HISTOLOGICAL DIFFERENTIAL

1. Dermatofibroma:
- Less fascicular
- Rounder and more polymorphic cells
- Foamy macrophages may be present
- Epidermal hyperplasia
2. Leiomyosarcoma:
- Presence of nuclear atypia
- Mitotic figures, some of them atypical
- Necrosis

SPECIAL STUDIES

- Immunohistochemistry with antibodies against smooth muscle actin or desmin

CLINICAL VARIANTS

- Piloleiomyoma
- Genital leiomyoma
- Angioleiomyoma

IMPORTANT THINGS TO KNOW

- Differentiation between piloleimyomas and genital leiomyomas is significant for prognosis: patients with multiple dermal leiomyomas experience recurrence at 50% rate, while patients with genital leiomyomas usually remain disease-free up to 5 years of follow up

Introduction

Leiomyosarcoma is a malignant tumor composed of cells showing distinct smooth muscle differentiation. Primary cutaneous leiomyosarcomas are infrequent tumors that may arise in the dermis or subcutaneous tissue. Secondary leiomyosarcomas are exceedingly rare. Dermal and subcutaneous lesions have a different biological behavior.

Histological features

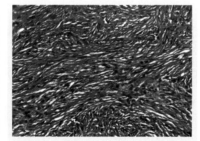

1. Flattening of the rete ridges
2. Interlacing fascicles of cells
3. Elongated spindle-shaped cells with eosinophilic cytoplasm and eccentric, blunt (cigar-shaped) nuclei
4. Multinucleated cells
5. Small lymphoid aggregates
6. Infiltrative margins
7. Moderate to severe cytological atypia and necrosis

Other features:
- More than 5 mitoses/10 high-power fields (HPF)

Leiomyosarcoma

Histological differential

1. Dermatofibrosarcoma protuberans:
- Widely infiltrative and monotonous cells
- Storiform pattern
2. Leiomyomas:
- Centered in reticular dermis but may extend into surrounding fat, tissue, or subcutis
- Poorly circumscribed fascicles of smooth muscle and collagen

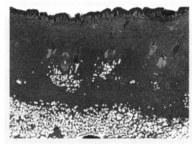

Dermatofibrosarcoma protuberans   Leiomyoma

Important Things To Know

- Dermal leiomyosarcomas may recur locally in up to 30% of cases. The recurrence rate seems to be lower when wide surgical excision is carried out initially
- Subcutaneous leiomyosarcomas tend to be slightly larger and more circumscribed. They have a greater tendency for local recurrence (50–70%), and metastases to lung, liver, and other sites

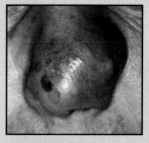

Epidemiology

- Soft tissue leiomyosarcoma usually occurs in middle-aged or older persons, although it may develop in young adults and even in children
- Predilection for the extensor surfaces of the extremities, and to a lesser extent the scalp, and trunk
- There is a male predominance

Pathophysiology

- Primary cutaneous leiomyosarcomas are infrequent tumors that may arise in the dermis or subcutaneous tissue
- Dermal tumors presumably arise from the erector pili muscles, except for scrotal lesions, which derive from the dartos muscle
- Subcutaneous leiomyosarcomas arise from the smooth muscle in vessel walls
- The most frequent genomic alterations in leiomyosarcomas involve losses in the 13q4–q21 region

Clinical features

- Presents as a mass lesion. The tumors vary in size from 0.5–3 cm or more in maximum diameter. Subcutaneous extension is present in two-thirds of cases
- Pain or tenderness is present in some
- Other symptoms depend on location

Special studies

- Immunoperoxidase preparations show the presence of vimentin, smooth muscle actin, and H-caldesmon

Clinical Variants

- Retroperitoneal sarcomas
- Limb sarcomas

NEURAL TUMORS

NERVE SHEATH TUMORS • NEUROFIBROMA

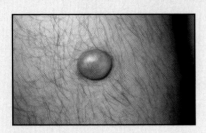

EPIDEMIOLOGY

- Solitary cutaneous lesions are common in young adults and have no gender preference
- Plexiform NF almost always indicate NF1

PATHOPHYSIOLOGY

- Neurofibromas are a complex proliferation of neuromesenchymal tissue, which includes Schwann cells, perineural cells, endoneural cells, and mast cells
- With NF1 associated neurofibromas, genetic studies have indicated mutations in the *NF1* gene cause inactivation of the neurofibroma protein or haplo insufficiency

CLINICAL FEATURES

- Clinically, neurofibromas are most commonly seen in the second and third decade of life, they are ill-defined, soft, asymptomatic skin-colored to tan papules or nodules ranging in size from 0.2–2.0 cm
- Plexiform neurofibromas are most commonly seen in the limbs, where they may be seen as huge pendulous masses causing deformity, which in extreme cases are known as elephantiasis neurofibromatosa. There is almost always associated osseous hypertrophy in the bony structures underneath these masses

SPECIAL STUDIES

- Immunohistochemically, the neoplastic cells stain positive with antibodies against the S-100 protein and Leu-7
- Occasionally neurites are also found within neurofibromas, which can be demonstrated using antibodies against neurofilament
- CD34 is sometimes focally positive

CLINICAL VARIANTS

- Neurofibromatosis type 1 and 2

INTRODUCTION

Neurofibromas (NF) can be classified either as solitary or multiple. Solitary NF are incidental findings and are usually not associated with systemic manifestations. Multiple NF on the other hand may be seen in patients with neurofibromatosis or von Recklinhausen's disease.

HISTOLOGICAL FEATURES

1. Well-circumscribed, non-encapsulated lesions involving the dermis and subcutaneous tissue
2. Composed of spindle cells with wavy nuclei and indistinct cytoplasmic borders
3. The stroma has variable amounts of mucin-containing mast cells

Other features:
- Small nerve fibers
- Varying amounts of collagen are present and sometimes there is a marked myxoid stroma

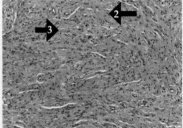

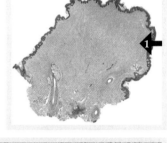

NEUROFIBROMA

HISTOLOGICAL DIFFERENTIAL

1. Schwannoma:
- Encapsulated
- Antoni A and Antoni B areas
- Verocay bodies
- Sclerotic vessels
2. Palisaded and encapsulate neuroma:
- Usually in the face
- Well-circumscribed lesions with clefts inside the neoplasm
- No myxoid stroma

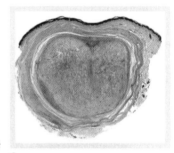

SCHWANNOMA

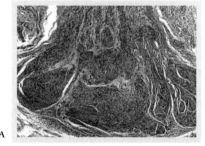

PALISADED AND ENCAPSULATED NEUROMA

IMPORTANT THINGS TO KNOW

- Plexiform neurofibroma carries a higher probability of malignant transformation (2–13%)

Schwannoma (neurilemmoma)

Introduction

Schwannomas or neurilemmomas are benign encapsulated neoplasms that can affect any anatomical site but are preferentially found in the head, neck and extremities. In contrast to neurofibromas these neoplasms are not associated with neurofibromatosis.

Histological features

1. Well-circumscribed nodules, surrounded by a capsule formed by perineurium
2. Two different areas which in some foci are imperceptibly merged:
   a. Antoni A
   b. Antoni B

- Antoni A areas have increased cellularity of spindle cells with wavy nuclei, slightly granular cytoplasm and indistinctive borders. In some foci the nuclei have a palisaded arrangement (Verocay bodies), a characteristic feature of schwannomas
- Antoni B areas are less cellular and are formed by a myxoid stroma containing dilated vessels, some of which have thick, sclerotic walls and Schwann cells

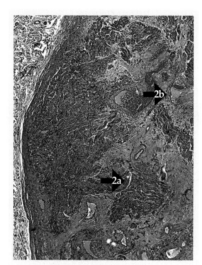

SCHWANNOMA

Histological variants:
- Cellular schwannoma: well-circumscribed, symmetrical, encapsulated neoplasms with increased cellularity and more atypia than regular schwannomas, occasional mitotic figures, but behave in a benign fashion
- Ancient schwannoma: characterized by cytologic atypia and degenerative changes including cystic areas, calcifications, hemorrhage with thromboses, thick vessels with sclerotic walls, xanthomatous areas, fibrosis, siderophages and atypical cells with bizarre, pleomorphic nuclei
- Plexiform schwannoma: lesion formed by multiple, well-delimited nodules, separated by fibrous tissue
- Most of these nodules are composed of Antoni A areas with a variable number of Verocay bodies. Antoni B areas are fewer or absent. Plexiform schwannomas are not associated with either malignant transformation or with von Recklinhausen's disease
- Psammomatous melanocytic schwannoma (PMS): associated with Carney's syndrome and can be multiple. It is well circumscribed and is less likely encapsulated than classic schwannoma. It shows heavily pigmented dendritic melanocytes. The melanin is produced by the neoplastic cells. Psammoma bodies are found in varying number. Occasionally they can metastasize causing death of the patients

Epidemiology

- More common in women with onset at age 20–50 years
- Uncommon disease
- 90% are solitary lesions
- Unknown etiology, possible link to *NF2* gene
- Occasionally associated with meningiomas or neurofibromatosis

Pathophysiology

- The tumor results from the proliferation of Schwann cells of peripheral nerve sheath derivation
- Mutations in the *NF2* gene, located at 22q12.2 is characteristic of vestibular schwannomas and other tumors; and in (familial) schwannomatosis

Clinical features

- The tumor is gray–white in color, encapsulated, with a smooth, glistening appearance, measuring 2–4 cm in diameter
- Cystic change is sometimes present, particularly in the larger, deeper tumors
- Slow-growing, usually solitary tumors with a propensity for the limbs of adults
- Pain, tenderness, and paresthesia may be present in up to one-third of lesions

Special studies

- Immunohistochemically schwannomas stain strongly with the S-100 protein, collagen type IV and Leu-7
- No axons can be demonstrated in these lesions

Important Things To Know

- Recurrence and malignant transformation are exceedingly rare

Clinical Variants

- Solitary, plexiform schwannomas
- Psammomatous melanocytic schwannoma (associated with Carney's syndrome)

HISTOLOGICAL DIFFERENTIAL

1. Palisaded and encapsulated neuroma:
- Well-circumscribed neoplasm
- No capsule
- Usually located on the face
- No Verocay bodies
2. Angioleiomyoma:
- Smooth muscle cells with blunt-ended nuclei and more eosinophilic cytoplasm

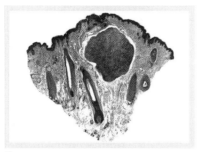

PALISADED AND ENCAPSULATED NEUROMA

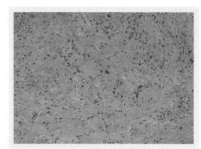

ANGIOLEIOMYOMA

SCHWANNOMA VARIANTS

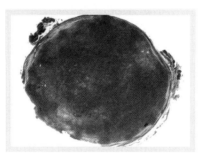

CELLULAR SCHWANNOMA

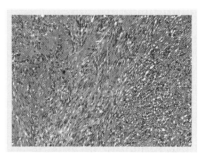

CELLULAR SCHWANNOMA

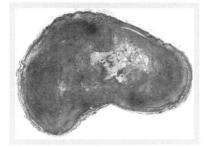

ANCIENT SCHWANNOMA

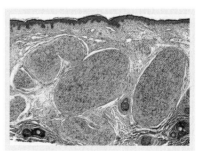

PLEXIFORM SCHWANNOMA

PSAMMOMATOUS MELANOCYTIC SCHWANNOMA

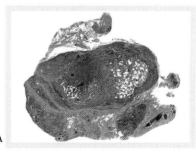

PERINEURIOMA

INTRODUCTION

Perineurioma is a rare benign neural neoplasm, composed exclusively of peri-neurial cells. It was originally described as presenting in the subcutaneous tissue as soft tissue perineurioma or storiform perineural fibroma.

HISTOLOGICAL FEATURES

1. Well-circumscribed tumor
2. Bland, short, spindle-shaped cells arranged in fascicles, with a focal whorling and a storiform pattern

Other features:
- Tumor cells may have epithelioid morphology
- Variable hyalinization of the collagen is present and some cases show scattered, mononuclear inflammatory cells
- Histological variants: intraneural, sclerosing, soft tissue, malignant

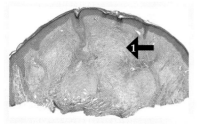
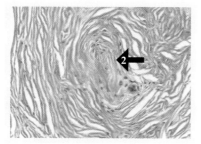

PERINEURIOMA

HISTOLOGICAL DIFFERENTIAL

1. Acquired digital fibrokeratoma:
- Admixture of prominent fibroblasts and vessels
- Negative for EMA
2. Neuroma:
- Lack a storiform pattern
- Generally S-100 protein positive
3. Infantile digital fibroma:
- Proliferation of fibroblasts with characteristic cytoplasmic inclusions
- Inclusions positive for vimentin and phosphotungstin hematoxylin

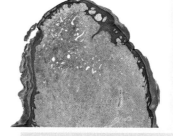

ACQUIRED DIGITAL FIBROKERATOMA

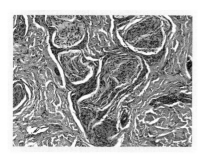

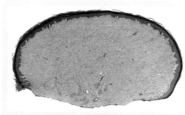

INFANTILE DIGITAL FIBROMA

NEUROMA

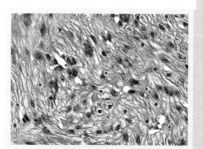

INFANTILE DIGITAL FIBROMA

EPIDEMIOLOGY

- Cutaneous perineurioma is relatively common
- Found mainly on the lower limbs of middle-aged adults
- Predilection for females

PATHOPHYSIOLOGY

- Unknown

CLINICAL FEATURES

- Presents as a small papular lesion, mainly on the lower limbs of middle-aged adults

SPECIAL STUDIES

- Tumor cells are diffusely positive for EMA, claudin, and Glut-1, but negative for other neural markers (including S-100 protein), in keeping with perineurial differentiation

IMPORTANT THINGS TO KNOW

- Soft tissue perineurioma has very similar clinical features to those of cutaneous variants but lesions are subcutaneous and tend to be larger (up to 5 cm)
- Behavior is benign with no tendency for local recurrence
- Malignant soft tissue perineuriomas are exceptional

CLINICAL VARIANTS

- None

EPIDEMIOLOGY

- Affects equally both males and females and it is more common in adults

PATHOPHYSIOLOGY

- Some of these cases occur predominantly on the face and are associated with acne-like changes, suggesting that minor trauma may play a role in their histogenesis

CLINICAL FEATURES

- Solitary well-circumscribed papules usually on the face, but they can also be seen in the buccal, nasal, or genital mucosa
- These lesions are most of time confused with melanocytic nevi or basal cell carcinomas

SPECIAL STUDIES

- Positive for S-100
- Variable number of axons, which stain positive for neurofilament protein

CLINICAL VARIANTS

- None

PALISADED AND ENCAPSULATED NEUROMAS

INTRODUCTION

Palisaded and encapsulated neuromas (PENs) clinically presents as solitary, small hemispheric papules color skin and usually localized to the face.

HISTOLOGICAL FEATURES

1. Well-circumscribed lesion made up of fascicles of nerve fibers and Schwann cells
2. Small clefts separating the fascicles of neoplastic cells and the surrounding stroma (a characteristic finding)
3. Appearance of the encapsulation due to a compression of the perilesional collagen fibers due to the expansile growth of the neoplasm

Other features:
- In some cases, the nuclei of the neoplastic cells showed a palisaded array
- Histopathological variants of PEN, include plexiform and epithelioid variants

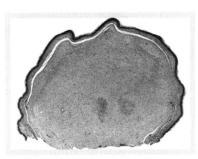 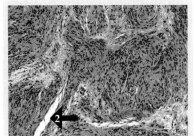

PALISADED AND ENCAPSULATED NEUROMA

HISTOLOGICAL DIFFERENTIAL

1. Neurofibroma:
- Not as circumscribed as PEN
- No clefts inside the tumor
2. Schwannoma:
- Well-circumscribed lesion surrounded by perineurium
- Verocay bodies
- EMA positivity at the periphery of the lesion

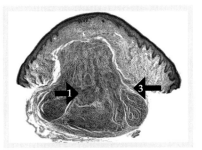 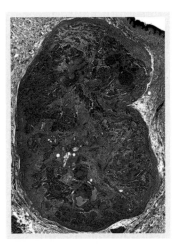

NEUROFIBROMA

SCHWANNOMA

IMPORTANT THINGS TO KNOW

- Occasionally PEN may present with multiple lesions

Cutaneous ganglioneuroma

Introduction

Cutaneous ganglioneuroma is a rare entity with only a few cases described so far.

Histological features

1. Ganglion cells, which are large with a round to star shape, prominent vesiculous nuclei, and cytoplasm filled with granules (Nissl substance)
2. Randomly distributed fusiform cells, embedded in a myxoid matrix

Other features:
- Nerve fibers may be found in the deeper parts of the lesion

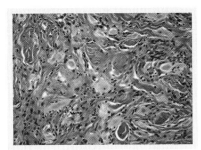

CUTANEOUS GANGLIONEUROMA

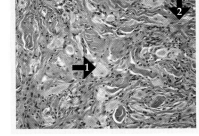

CUTANEOUS GANGLIONEUROMA

Histological differential

1. Cutaneous metastasis of neuroblastoma:
- Clinical data is helpful

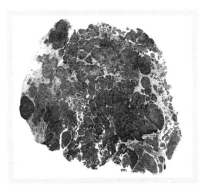

NEUROBLASTOMA

Epidemiology

- Affects both males and females
- No age preference
- More common in the trunk and rarely affects the face and limbs

Pathophysiology

- This lesion is a hamartoma and results from abnormal migration of ganglion and Schwann cell precursors, which are derived from the neural crest to the skin

Clinical features

- Clinically, these lesions appear as papules, nodules or pedunculated lesions

Special studies

- Ganglion cells stain with neurofilament, neuron-specific enolase, synaptophysin and glial fibrillary acidic protein, but do not stain with S-100 while the fusiform cells are intensely positive for this marker

Important Things To Know

- Rare entity with only a few cases described to date

Clinical Variants

- None

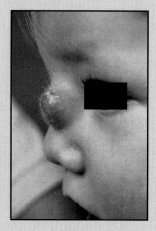

EPIDEMIOLOGY

- May be present at birth or develop during the first months of life
- No gender predilection

PATHOPHYSIOLOGY

- Nasal gliomas may be considered small encephaloceles caused by trapping of glial tissue within subcutaneous tissue during early embryonic development

CLINICAL FEATURES

- NGs are situated either at the root of the nose or intranasally, or in both sites concurrently
- When the latter occurs, communication exits between the intranasal and extranasal parts usually through a defect in the middle of the nasal bone or at its lateral margin
- 20% of nasal gliomas are connected to the brain by a pedicle of glial tissue. For this reason, before manipulating a nasal glioma it is important to establish that there is no connection with the brain, to avoid complications such as infections or cerebrospinal liquid leakage. In most cases they are single lesions, with multiple neoplasms being found only rarely

SPECIAL STUDIES

- Strongly positive for vimentin, S-100 protein, CD57, and glial fibrillary acidic protein

CLINICAL VARIANTS

- Encephaloceles

NASAL GLIOMA

INTRODUCTION

Nasal gliomas (NGs) are rare, slowly growing choristomas that are detected early in infancy or childhood, and are localized to the nasofrontal region. They are composed of glial tissue with occasional neurons

HISTOLOGICAL FEATURES

1. Ill-defined neoplasm of variable size that involve the dermis and subcutaneous tissue
2. Groups of astrocytes with pale, fibrillary and/or granular cytoplasm and a centrally placed nucleus
3. No pleomorphism and no mitotic figures are noticeable
4. The collections of astrocytes are separated from one another by variable amounts of collagen

Other features:
- Sometimes there are prominent multinucleated cells, associated with abundant pale cytoplasm
- No typical neurons are usually identified, but a prominent neuronal component has been described
- Encephaloceles, which are rare, congenital, cystic malformations, may be considered to be the cystic variant of NG. The cavity of the cyst is usually filled with cerebrospinal fluid and blood, and is lined by a thin layer of ependymal cells. The wall of the cyst is formed by glial tissue and skin. The glial tissue is histologically similar to that seen in nasal gliomas. Encephaloceles are connected usually to the brain and cerebral ventricles by a stalk of glial tissue that extends through a defect in the cranium

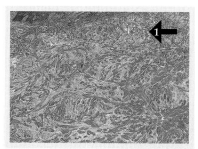

NASAL GLIOMA

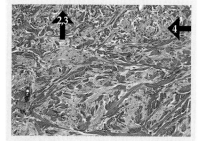

NASAL GLIOMAS

HISTOLOGICAL DIFFERENTIAL

1. Meningothelial hamartoma:
- Small collections of meningothelial cells
- Pseudovascular spaces
- No psammoma bodies

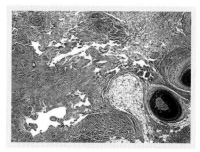

MENINGOTHELIAL HAMARTOMA

IMPORTANT THINGS TO KNOW

- In some cases there are communications with the frontal lobe, this communication must be interrupted before excision of the skin lesion

Cutaneous meningioma

Introduction

Meningiomas, are among the most common neoplasms in the central nervous system, and are characterized by their sharp circumscription and benign behavior. These neoplasms are rarely found in locations other than the central nervous system and when they are, it is usually in the orbit or the skin. There are three types of meningiomas: type I or congenital meningiomas; type II meningiomas are localized near sensory organs; and type III meningiomas that are extensions from the central nervous system.

Histological features

1. Symmetrical and well-circumscribed benign neoplasms involving dermis and sometimes extending into subcutaneous tissue
2. Nests and clusters of cells arranged in whorls. Cells are in a syncytial arrangement

Other features:
- The epidermis is spared
- Laminated formations with or without calcification (psammoma bodies)
- An uncommon type of cutaneous meningiomas is the so-called angioblastic meningioma or meningothelial hamartoma. This neoplasm is typified by prominent pseudovascular spaces, which cause it to resemble a vascular neoplasm
- The three types of meningiomas are very similar to one another histopathologically, although type II and III meningiomas are associated with a variable number of inflammatory cells, whereas the congenital type of meningioma (type I) is devoid of inflammatory cells

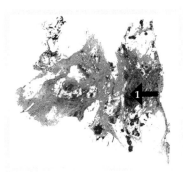 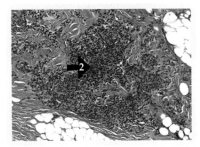

CUTANEOUS MENINGIOMA

Histological differential

1. Cellular neurothekeoma:
- Irregular collections of epithelioid cells which anastomose with each other
- Lobular pattern of growth
- S-100 negative, positive for NK1-C3 (CD63)
- Cells with abundant amphophilic cytoplasm with ill-defined cell borders

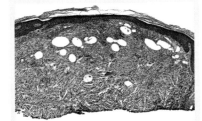

CELLULAR NEUROTHEKEOMA

IMPORTANT THINGS TO KNOW

- It must be emphasized that cutaneous meningiomas are sometimes directly connected to the central nervous system. Extreme caution needs to be taken, in their manipulation because complications such as meningitis may result

Epidemiology

- Most commonly seen in children and young adults, but may appear at any age
- Usually on the scalp, face, or in the paraspinal region
- They may present either as solitary or multiple neoplasms

Pathophysiology

- Congenital meningiomas result from failure in the closure of the neural tube during embryonic development
- Meningiomas localized to near sensory organs results of remnants of arachnoidal tissue entrapped in the neural sheaths of cranial or spinal nerves
- Type III meningiomas are extensions of meningiomas that originated in the central nervous system

Clinical features

- These neoplasms may be either firm or soft, and may have digitated projections
- There are differences between three types of meningiomas:
  o Type I represents congenital meningiomas result in the presence of ectopic meningeal tissue in the dermis and subcutaneous fat. This variant has good prognosis and most commonly occurs on the scalp, forehead, and paravertebral region
  o Type II comprises meningiomas localized to near sensory organs, such as the eye and ear, and involve the skin by continuity. Type II meningiomas produce symptoms that depend upon the sensory organ involved (e.g. proptosis and periorbital edema when positioned near an eye, or tympanomastoiditis when situated within or near the temporal bone)
  o Type III meningiomas involve the skin through surgical defects, erosion of the cranial vault or metastasis to the skin

Special studies

- Usually positive for vimentin and EMA, D2-40/podoplanin
- Positivity for S-100 is variable

Clinical Variants

- None

EPIDEMIOLOGY

- Most commonly in the skin and tongue
- In most cases they are single entities
- Mainly affect people in the third to the fifth decade of life
- More common in women than in men

PATHOPHYSIOLOGY

- Immunohistochemical and ultrastructural studies have demonstrated the schwannian lineage of tumor cells in granular cell tumor

CLINICAL FEATURES

- They present as small, firm masses, either sessile or pedunculated, with ill-defined margins
- The color varies from pink to greyish brown
- The overlying epidermis may be hyperkeratotic or verrucous and is sometimes ulcerated which may lead to their being confused with malignant neoplasms

SPECIAL STUDIES

- Positive staining with the S-100 protein
- PAS is positive

CLINICAL VARIANTS

- None

GRANULAR CELL TUMOR

INTRODUCTION

Granular cell tumors (GCT) are a group of neoplasms named for their distinctive appearance under the light microscope. They are characterized by the presence of cells with large, granular and eosinophilic cytoplasm. GCT is an asymptomatic, slow-growing neoplasm and is usually an incidental finding. Most authors agree that GCT, especially those localized in the mouth and the skin, have neural differentiation.

HISTOLOGICAL FEATURES

1. Small, poorly circumscribed neoplasm present in the dermis and occasionally in the subcutaneous tissue
2. Pseudoepitheliomatous hyperplasia
3. Nests or strands of pale-staining, round to polygonal cells with a centrally placed, small nucleus and faintly eosinophilic cytoplasmic granules
4. The stroma composed of connective tissue

Other features:
- Older lesions may show prominent desmoplasia with few granular cells

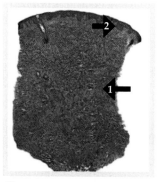

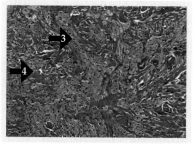

GRANULAR CELL TUMOR

GRANULAR CELL TUMOR

HISTOLOGICAL DIFFERENTIAL

1. Dermatofibroma:
- Proliferation of fibroblasts admixed with kelloidal collagen
- Presence of multinucleated cells occasionally
- S-100 negative and Factor XIII positive
2. Leiomyoma:
- Proliferation of fascicles of smooth muscle cells intersecting with each other
- Actin, desmin positive, S-100 negative

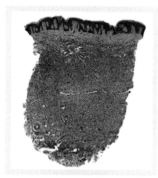

DERMATOFIBROMA

IMPORTANT THINGS TO KNOW

- In superficial biopsies, GCT can be confused with squamous cell carcinoma because of the degree of epidermal hyperplasia

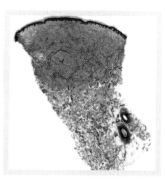

LEIOMYOMA

VASCULAR TUMORS

HYPERPLASIAS • PYOGENIC GRANULOMA

INTRODUCTION

Pyogenic granuloma (PG) is a hyperplastic process. The lesion grows rapidly at sites of superficial trauma. In some cases lesions of PG are associated to endocrine alterations or medication and usually involute upon cessation of the stimuli.

HISTOLOGICAL FEATURES

1. Fully developed lesions of PG are polypoid and show a lobular pattern with fibrous septa intersecting the lesion
2. Each lobule is composed of aggregations of capillaries and venules lined by plump endothelial cells
3. Pale edematous stroma

Other features:
• Early lesions of PG are identical to granulation tissue, to wit, numerous capillaries and venules disposed radially to the skin surface, which is often eroded and covered with scabs

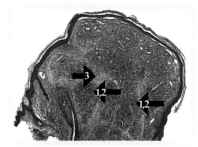
PYOGENIC GRANULOMA

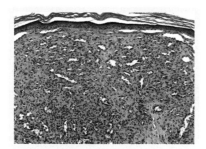
PYOGENIC GRANULOMA

HISTOLOGICAL DIFFERENTIAL

1. Hemangioma:
• No edema and prominent septa
• No inflammation
2. Bacillary angiomatosis:
• More neutrophils
• Purple cytoplasmic inclusions in endothelial cells which represent bacilli

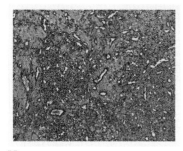
HEMANGIOMA

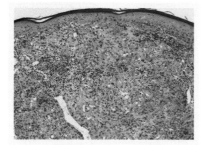
BACILLARY ANGIOMATOSIS

IMPORTANT THINGS TO KNOW
• Intravascular PG appears as a PG inside of a vein

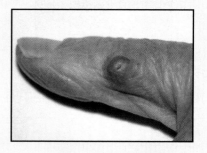

EPIDEMIOLOGY
• Can develop at any age, but is more common in children and young adults

PATHOPHYSIOLOGY
• Majority of the cases have no apparent cause, a minority follow trauma or retinoid therapy
• Hormonal factors may be involved in their genesis

CLINICAL FEATURES
• Affects both the skin and mucous membranes
• Rapidly growing solitary red friable papule or nodule
• May develop following minor trauma
• Occurs most often on an exposed surface

SPECIAL STUDIES
• The vascular markers CD31, CD34 and factor VIII are positive

CLINICAL VARIANTS
• Cutaneous
• Mucosal
• Solitary
• Multicentric

INFANTILE HEMANGIOMAS

INTRODUCTION

Infantile hemangioma is the most common benign vascular proliferation, and traditionally has been considered a neoplasm. The majority of these lesions, after an initial proliferative phase, undergo complete regression through a process of fibrosis, even in the absence of therapy. True neoplastic infantile hemangiomas include noninvoluting congenital hemangiomas (NICH) and rapidly involuting congenital nonhemangiomas (RICH). These two lesions do not regress as do the other infantile hemangiomas

HISTOLOGICAL FEATURES

1. Early hemangiomas are highly cellular and are characterized by plump endothelial cells aligned to vascular spaces with small inconspicuous lumina
- The histopathological composition of infantile hemangiomas varies with the age of the lesion
- As the lesions mature, blood flow increases, endothelium flattens, and the lumina of the vessels enlarge and become more obvious
- During this interval the vessels convey a "cavernous" appearance that can be misinterpreted as a venous malformation. Regression is portrayed as progressive interstitial fibrosis and adipose metaplasia, a process without known stimulus

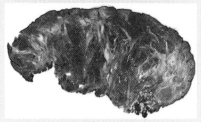 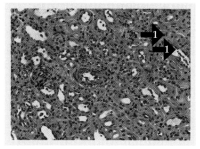

INFANTILE HEMANGIOMA

HISTOLOGICAL DIFFERENTIAL

1. Pyogenic granuloma (PG):
- PG is often ulcerated and has edema and inflammation

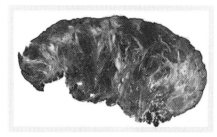

PYOGENIC GRANULOMA

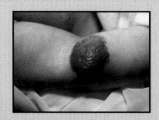

EPIDEMIOLOGY

- The most common tumors of infancy, with an incidence in the newborn population of approximately 2%
- There is a female preponderance

PATHOPHYSIOLOGY

- A locus for autosomal dominant predisposition to hemangiomas has been identified on chromosome 5q
- Ischemic placental injuries are associated with an increase in infantile hemangiomas

CLINICAL FEATURES

- Infantile hemangioma is the most common tumor of infancy. It is usually not present at birth but becomes apparent within first few weeks of life and is more common in premature infants. The majority of lesions regress by 5-7 years of age
- Usually bright red to blue papule, nodule, or plaque varying in size from a few millimeters to several centimeters

SPECIAL STUDIES

- GLUT-1+, WT1+, CD31+ are positive in classical infantile hemangiomas
- GUT-1 is negative in NICH and RICH

CLINICAL VARIANTS

- Rapidly involuting congenital hemangioma (RICH)
- Non-involuting congenital hemangioma (NICH)

IMPORTANT THINGS TO KNOW

- Glut-1 allows discrimination between classical infantile hemangiomas, RICH, and NICH

CHERRY ANGIOMAS

INTRODUCTION

Senile or cherry angiomas, known also as Campbell de Morgan spots are among the most frequently acquired cutaneous vascular lesions.

HISTOLOGICAL FEATURES

1. Cherry angioma consists of dilated capillary blood vessels localized in the superficial dermis
2. The vessels have variably thickened walls
3. Fully developed lesions are associated with a loss of the rete ridges of the epidermis that leads to the formation of a peripheral collarette of adnexal epithelium, thus creating a polypoid lesion

Other features:

- Mast cells may be numerous, while the endothelial cells that line the vessels express a strong carbonic anhydrase activity, as a correlate with the fenestration of the venous capillaries

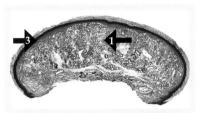 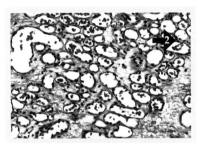

CHERRY HEMANGIOMA

HISTOLOGICAL DIFFERENTIAL

1. Angiosarcoma:
- Poor circumscription
- Irregular vascular spaces which anastomose with each other
- Atypical endothelial cells

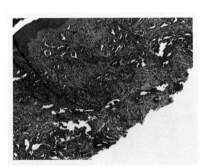

ANGIOSARCOMA

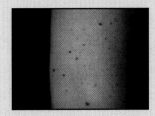

EPIDEMIOLOGY

- They appear early in adulthood, most commonly on the trunk and lower extremities with time, may increase in number and size

PATHOPHYSIOLOGY

- Some authors have suggested that cherry angiomas may be related to a recent rise in the atmospheric temperature, since the number of lesions per patient increased and decreased proportionate to the temperature
- Eruptive cherry hemangiomas have also been concurrent with ECHO viral infections, as well as exposures to chemical compounds, notably glycol ether solvent 2-butoxyethanol, sulfur mustard gas, and bromides

CLINICAL FEATURES

- They appear early in adulthood, most commonly on the trunk and proximal limbs and with time, may increase in number and size. On presentation they are small red papules that resist compression

SPECIAL STUDIES

- Proliferation activity is very low, as expressed negatively by an absence of immunohistochemical reactivity for Ki67
- CD31 and CD34 positivity in the endothelial cells

IMPORTANT THINGS TO KNOW

- Hormonal factors have also been suspect. It has been observed that pregnant women are disposed during pregnancy with lesions that involutes post-partum

CLINICAL VARIANTS

- None

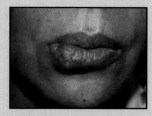

Epidemiology

- Arteriovenous hemangioma is a neoplasm that occurs in mid-adult life

Pathophysiology

- The precise nature of acral arteriovenous hemangioma is uncertain
- Some of studies proposed that it is a multicentric hamartoma of the subpapillary vascular plexus with one or more arteriovenous anastomosis

Clinical features

- It presents as a blue to red papule measuring 0.5–1.0 cm, mainly affecting facial skin
- Larger lesions as well as intraoral and vulvar examples have been also described
- Usually the lesions are solitary, although multiple examples have been cited
- When the lesions are multiple they tend to cluster together
- Occasionally, they are associated with other abnormalities including epidermal nevus syndrome, vascular hamartomas and malformations; and several examples of multiple arteriovenous hemangiomas have been described in patients with chronic liver disease

Special studies

- None

Clinical Variants

- None

Arteriovenous hemangioma

Introduction

This lesion was first named cirsoid aneurysm, because of the presence of a spiraled blood vessel (feeder vessel) extending from the subcutaneous fat into the lesion. Recently, it was renamed arteriovenous hemangioma or acral arteriovenous tumor. The latter name is not totally appropriate, because this lesion affects different areas of the body and not only acral skin.

Histological features

1. Well-circumscribed proliferation of thick-walled muscle-containing blood vessels, lined by a single layer of endothelial cells involving the upper and mid-reticular dermis
2. There are also thin-walled dilated blood vessels
3. Spiraled ascending small muscular artery ("feeder" vessel)

Other features:
- The thick-walled blood vessels resemble arteries, but a well-formed elastic internal membrane is absent. Therefore, they are probably ectatic veins
- Arteriovenous shunts

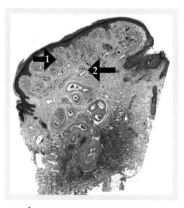
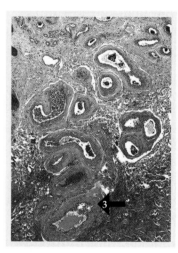

ARTERIOVENOUS HEMANGIOMA

Histological differential

1. Glomangioma:
- Large dilated blood vessels surrounded by several layer of cuboidal cells

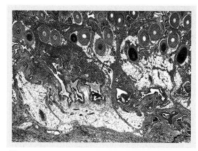
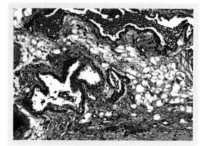

GLOMANGIOMA

GLOMANGIOMA

Microvenular hemangioma

Introduction

Microvenular hemangioma is a recently described benign vascular neoplasm.

Histological features

1. Poorly circumscribed proliferation of irregularly branched, round to oval, thin-walled blood vessels lined by a single layer of endothelial cells, involving the entire reticular dermis
2. The lumina of the neoplastic blood vessels are inconspicuous and often collapse with only a few erythrocytes within them
3. Variable degree of dermal sclerosis in the stroma

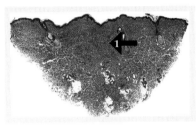
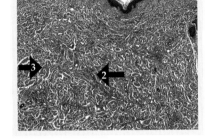

MICROVENULAR HEMANGIOMA

Histological differential

1. Kaposi sarcoma, patch stage:
- Irregular anastomosing vascular spaces
- Newly formed ectatic vascular channels surrounding pre-existing normal blood vessels and adnexa (promontory sign)
- Plasma cells
- Hyaline (eosinophilic) globules
- Small interstitial fascicles of spindle cells

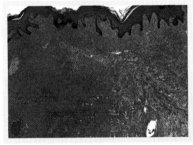

KAPOSI SARCOMA, PATCH STAGE

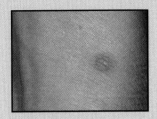

Epidemiology

- Affects males and females equally

Pathophysiology

- In some patients, a histogenetic relationship between microvenular hemangioma and hormonal factors, such as pregnancy and hormonal contraceptives, has been postulated, but this feature has not been corroborated by other authors

Clinical features

- Microvenular hemangioma is an acquired, slowly growing asymptomatic lesion with angiomatous appearance
- It is usually solitary, varying in size from 0.5–2 cm
- It most commonly affects the upper limbs, particularly the forearms. However, lesions on the trunk, face and lower limbs have also been recorded
- Hemangiomas identical to microvenular hemangioma can be seen in patients with POEMS syndrome

Special studies

- Immunohistochemically, the cells lining the lumina show positivity for factor VIII-related antigen, CD31 and CD34 which qualifies them as endothelial cells
- Some smooth muscle actin-positive perithelial cells have been also described surrounding this vascular space

Important things to know

- Lesions of microvenular hemangioma are cured by simple excision

Clinical variants

- None

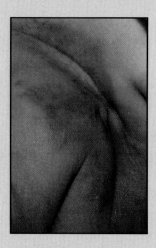

EPIDEMIOLOGY

- Most commonly affect children and young adults, but both congenital and very late onset cases have been described

PATHOPHYSIOLOGY

- Most cases are sporadic, although a family with several members affected by tufted angioma has been reported. In this particular family the mode of transmission was in an autosomal dominant fashion

CLINICAL VARIANTS

- None

TUFTED ANGIOMA

INTRODUCTION

Tufted angioma is an unusual, acquired vascular neoplasm.

HISTOLOGICAL FEATURES

1. Multiple individual vascular lobules within the middle and lower dermis and subcutaneous fat
2. Aggregation of endothelial cells that whorl concentrically around a pre-existing vascular plexus in each lobule
3. The "cannon ball" pattern is characteristic of tufted angioma

Other features:
- Some lobules bulge into the walls of dilated thin-walled vascular structures, giving these vessels a slit-like or semilunar appearance
- Small capillary lumina are identified within the aggregations of endothelial cells

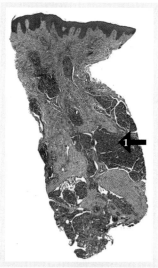

TUFTED ANGIOMA

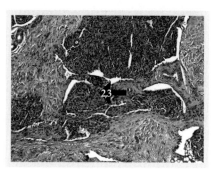

TUFTED ANGIOMA

HISTOLOGICAL DIFFERENTIAL

1. Kaposi sarcoma:
- Nodular lesions of Kaposi sarcoma are composed of interlacing fascicles of spindle cells lining slit-like vessels
- An inflammatory infiltrate of plasma cells is usually present
2. Infantile hemangiomas:
- Tufted angiomas are rare in infants
- Occasionally present with a lobular pattern, but these collections are present only focally

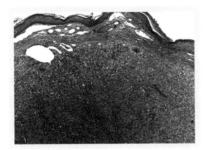

KAPOSI SARCOMA

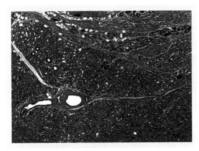

INFANTILE HEMANGIOMA

IMPORTANT THINGS TO KNOW

- Tufted angioma showing spontaneous regression is a rare event. For the treatment of these lesions, soft radiation has been recommended. Satisfactory results have been also reported with surgery, pulse-dye laser, high-dose of systemic steroids, and interferon-α

CLINICAL FEATURES

- The lesions have a predilection for the neck, upper chest, back, and shoulders, although examples of tufted angioma have also been reported on the head, extremities and oral mucosa
- Tufted angioma grows slowly and insidiously, and may eventually come to cover a large area of the trunk or neck. In most cases the growth is halted after some years, but there is a slight tendency toward spontaneous regression
- The clinical appearance of the lesions is variable. Some of them are characterized by enlarging erythematous or brown macules or plaques with an angiomatous appearance; other lesions may resemble granulomas or a connective tissue abnormality. In some cases the lesions are tender, while in other cases there is hyperhidrosis on the surface. Raised papules resembling pyogenic granulomas are sometimes seen within the area of the lesion and occasionally the lesions may show a linear arrangement
- Tufted angiomas have been associated with nevus flammeus and other vascular malformations, pregnancy, and with non-regressing lipodystrophy centrifugalis abdominalis. In some cases the lesion spread by infiltration, leading to sclerosing plaques. Many cases of Kasabach-Merritt syndrome are associated with tufted angioma

SPECIAL STUDIES

- The cells in the capillary tufts are weakly positive or negative for factor VIII-related antigen
- They exhibit strong positivity for Ulex europaeus I lectin, EN4, CD31, CD34 and alpha-smooth muscle actin which is related to the immature nature of the endothelial cells. The cells that show reactivity for smooth muscle actin, most likely represent pericytes

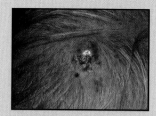

EPIDEMIOLOGY

- No sex predilection

PATHOPHYSIOLOGY

- Speculation remains as to the histogenesis of glomeruloid hemangioma. There is a hypothesis that the deposition of immunoglobulins within the endothelial cells stimulate the proliferation of these cells in a glomeruloid fashion

CLINICAL FEATURES

- Glomeruloid angiomas are small, firm, red to violaceous, dome-shaped papules that measure a few millimeters in diameter and are usually located on the trunk and proximal parts of the extremities
- In some cases the angiomatous lesions resemble eruptive histiocytomas

SPECIAL STUDIES

- The vacuoles in the cytoplasm of the endothelial cells contain eosinophilic PAS positive globules that represent deposits of immunoglobulins absorbed through circulation
- The neoplastic cells are positive for factor VIII-related antigen, Ulex europaeus I lectin and vimentin
- Muscle-specific actin is negative
- Two different types of endothelial cells have been described in glomeruloid hemangioma. The first type consists of endothelial cells with large vesicular nuclei with open chromatin and large amounts of cytoplasm. These cells are positive for CD31, CD34, and *Ulex europaeus I lectin*, but not for CD68. The second type of endothelial cells consists of cells with small nuclei containing a dense chromatin and scant cytoplasm. This second type of cells express positively for CD31 and CD68, whereas CD34 and *Ulex europaeus I lectin are negative*

CLINICAL VARIANTS

- None

GLOMERULOID HEMANGIOMA

INTRODUCTION

Glomeruloid hemangioma is a vascular proliferation that only occurs in patients affected with the POEMS syndrome. POEMS is an acronym for this syndrome which includes: Polyneuropathy, Organomegaly, Endocrinopathy, Monoclonal gammopathy (M protein), and Skin lesions. Histopathologically, the vascular lesion in patients with POEMS syndrome fall into four categories: microvenular hemangiomas; cherry hemangiomas; multinucleate cell angiohistiocytomas; and glomeruloid hemangiomas. Glomeruloid hemangiomas seem to be fairly specific for POEMS syndrome.

HISTOLOGICAL FEATURES

1. Multiple ectatic vascular structures containing aggregates of capillary loops resembling renal glomeruli
2. The capillaries are lined with either flat or plump endothelial cells with vacuoles and surrounded by pericytes

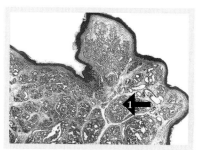
GLOMERULOID HEMANGIOMA

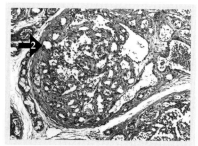
GLOMERULOID HEMANGIOMA

HISTOLOGICAL DIFFERENTIAL

1. Tufted angioma:
- Composed of solid aggregates of endothelial cells forming lobules, indenting dilated vessels
- Lack of glomeruloid arrangement
- No evidence of eosinophilic PAS positive deposits within the endothelial cells

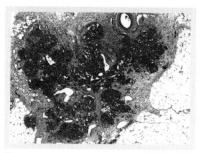
TUFTED ANGIOMA

IMPORTANT THINGS TO KNOW

- Most patients with POEMS syndrome have a progressive, disabling clinical course with a poor prognosis, in spite of any therapy

ACQUIRED ELASTOTIC HEMANGIOMA

INTRODUCTION

Acquired elastotic hemangioma is a recently described variant of cutaneous hemangioma. These lesions develop during adulthood on chronic sun-damaged skin, on the extensor surface of the forearms or the lateral aspects of the neck.

HISTOLOGICAL FEATURES

1. Band-like proliferation of capillaries involving only the superficial dermis
2. A narrow band of non-involved papillary dermis separates the newly formed capillaries from the normal or flattened epidermis
3. The neoformed capillaries show small cleft-like or round lumina and contain few erythrocytes
4. Solar elastosis in connective tissue surrounding or intermingled with the newly formed capillaries

Other features:
- No cellular atypia, no hemosiderin deposits or extravasated erythrocytes

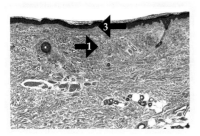

ACQUIRED ELASTOTIC HEMANGIOMA

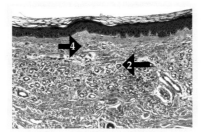

ACQUIRED ELASTOTIC HEMANGIOMA

HISTOLOGICAL DIFFERENTIAL

1. Angiosarcoma:
- Usually is located in head and neck, not arms
- Irregular proliferation of vessels, not capillaries
- Atypical endothelial cells throughout the dermis

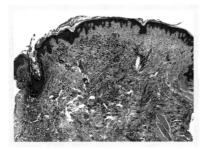

ANGIOSARCOMA

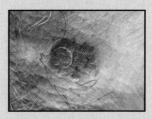

EPIDEMIOLOGY

- It mainly affects middle-aged and elderly women

PATHOPHYSIOLOGY

- Sun exposure appears to be an important factor in the development of these lesions

CLINICAL FEATURES

- Acquired elastotic hemangioma presents as a slightly elevated, irregularly shaped, solitary lesion with violaceous coloration
- The lesions are usually well-demarcated plaques that range from 2–5 cm in diameter
- The lesions blanch under diascope pressure

SPECIAL STUDIES

- The neoplastic endothelial cells are strongly positive for CD31 and CD34
- A continuous rim of alpha-smooth muscle actin-positive pericytes surrounds the majority of the neoplastic vascular channels
- Proliferating markers Ki-67 and MPM-2 stain only a few of the nuclei of the endothelial cells of the newly formed blood vessels

IMPORTANT THINGS TO KNOW

- Treatment consisted of local surgical excision in all cases

CLINICAL VARIANTS

- None

EPIDEMIOLOGY

- Most commonly affects children

PATHOPHYSIOLOGY

- When the neoplasm is positioned in deep soft tissue, mediastinum, or retroperitoneum, it may be associated with the consumption coagulopathy that characterizes Kasabach-Merritt syndrome
- In some cases, kaposiform hemangioendothelioma may be associated with lymphangiomatosis

CLINICAL FEATURES

- Affects the skin and also the retroperitoneum. Some patients may develop the Kasabach-Merritt syndrome

SPECIAL STUDIES

- Immunohistochemical studies have provided dissimilar results. In some cases the neoplastic cells were positive for vimentin, FLI-1, D2-40, CD31 and CD34 and negative for actin. In the better-formed vascular channels of the neoplasm, the latter marker highlights pericytes that form a ring around the negative stained endothelial cells. GLUT1 antibody is negative, but the vascular endothelial growth factor receptor-3 (VEGFR-3) has been reported positive in six cases studied, which suggests at least partial lymphatic endothelial differentiation of the neoplastic cells in kaposiform hemangioendothelioma. So far, no evidence of human herpes virus 8 (HHV-8) infection has been detected in lesions of kaposiform hemangioendothelioma

CLINICAL VARIANTS

- None

KAPOSIFORM HEMANGIOENDOTHELIOMA

INTRODUCTION

Kaposiform hemangioendothelioma is a rare vascular neoplasm. Though the retroperitoneum is the most frequent location, it may also be found in the skin.

HISTOLOGICAL FEATURES

1. Several ill-circumscribed nodules separated by connective tissue
2. Admixture of small round capillaries and solid glomeruloid nests containing round to oval endothelial cells with epithelioid features in nodules

Other features:
- The endothelial cells may contain hemosiderin, hyaline globules, and vacuoles
- Short fascicles of spindle cells within nodules
- Absence of atypia and mitotic figures

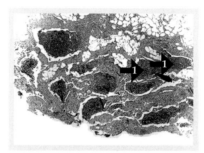
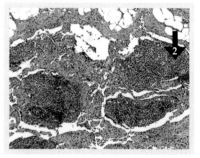

KAPOSIFORM HEMANGIOENDOTHELIOMA

HISTOLOGICAL DIFFERENTIAL

1. Tufted angioma:
- Nodules are smaller and more circumscribed
- Does not involve deep soft tissue or bone
2. Kaposi sarcoma:
- Absence of multinodular pattern
- Infiltrates of plasma cells present around the nodules

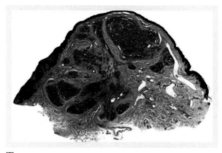
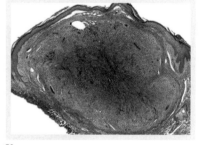

TUFTED ANGIOMA

KAPOSI SARCOMA

IMPORTANT THINGS TO KNOW

- Kaposiform hemangioendothelioma combines features of cellular infantile hemangioma and Kaposi sarcoma
- Kasabach-Merritt syndrome is a major complication of these lesions

GLOMUS TUMOR AND GLOMANGIOMA

INTRODUCTION

Glomus tumors are uncommon neoplasms that arise from modified smooth muscle cells normally present in specialized arteriovenous shunts in acral sites, mainly the fingertips.

HISTOLOGICAL FEATURES

Glomus tumor:

1. Well-circumscribed dermal tumor surrounded by compressed fibrous tissue
2. The neoplasm is cytologically formed of clusters of round or polygonal monomorphous glomus cells with large round, plump nuclei and scant eosinophilic cytoplasm

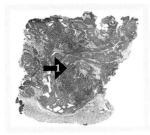 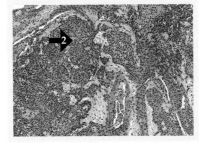

GLOMUS TUMOR

Glomangioma:

1. Less well-circumscribed lesions than solitary glomus tumors
2. These are composed of irregular dilated endothelial lined vascular channels that contain red blood cells and, distinctively have small intramural aggregations of glomus cells
- Some are made up of several nodules within the dermis
- Some have an appearance that calls to mind a hemangioma

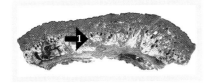

GLOMANGIOMA

GLOMANGIOMA

HISTOLOGICAL DIFFERENTIAL

1. Solid form of hidradenoma:
- Vascularity of glomus and lack of ductal differentiation help to differentiate
2. Venous malformation:
- Lack of glomus cells

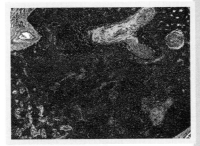

SOLID FORM OF HIDRADENOMA

IMPORTANT THINGS TO KNOW

- The tumor is positive for smooth muscle actin (SMA) and vimentin

EPIDEMIOLOGY

- Glomus tumor is more common in young adults
- Glomangioma is more common in infancy and childhood

PATHOPHYSIOLOGY

- Substance Present in nerve fibers has been incriminated in the pathophysiology of glomus tumors. This substance, it is known to be a primary sensory afferent neurotransmitter for mediating painful stimuli
- Multiple familial glomus tumors appear to have autosomal dominant pattern of inheritance

CLINICAL FEATURES

- The solitary glomus tumor is more common. It creates a small, purple nodule preferentially in acral areas of the extremities, especially nail beds of the fingers
- There is a striking predominance among female patients
- Frequently, the lesion creates severe paroxysmal pain, usually precipitated by exposure to cold or minor pressure
- In contrast to the solitary glomus lesion, glomangiomas present during childhood as small bluish nodules situated deep in the dermis and widely scattered in the skin

SPECIAL STUDIES

- SMA+, H-caldesmon+, Desmin, CD34, S-100 are negative

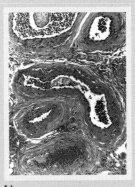

VENOUS MALFORMATION

CLINICAL VARIANTS

- Cutaneous
- Visceral

EPIDEMIOLOGY

- Classic Kaposi sarcoma affects elderly patients most frequently in males. A racial predisposition is recorded, with an increased incidence in Ashkenazi Jews and individuals of Mediterranean descent. It follows a chronic course and the lesions predominantly involve the lower parts of the legs
- The African-endemic variant of Kaposi sarcoma occurs mainly in equatorial Africa. This variant of Kaposi sarcoma has been subdivided into two groups:
  - o a benign nodular disease, affecting mainly young adults
  - o a fulminant lymphadenopathic form. This latter form is fatal, it predominantly affects children and kills most of the patients within two to three years
- The iatrogenic, immunosuppressive, drug-associated form of Kaposi sarcoma is especially frequent in renal transplant recipients, although it has also been reported in other organ transplant recipients, as well as in a wide spectrum of patients receiving immunosuppressive drug therapy for different reasons
- AIDS-associated Kaposi sarcoma is especially frequent in homosexual men, found in 21% of all homosexual men with AIDS

KAPOSI SARCOMA

INTRODUCTION

Vascular neoplasm caused by human herpes virus 8 (HHV-8).

HISTOLOGICAL FEATURES

1. Plaque lesions involve the entire dermis and even the upper part of the subcutaneous fat
2. At this stage, there is an increased number of spindle cells arranged in short fascicles between collagen bundles centered around proliferating vascular channels
3. The spindle cells line irregularly shaped, slit-like vascular spaces that contain isolated erythrocytes

Other features:
- The neoplastic vessels of Kaposi sarcoma show a tendency to be present around pre-existing normal adnexae and blood vessels producing the so-called "promontory sign"
- At scanning magnification patch stage lesions show sparse, superficial and deep perivascular mononuclear cell infiltrates in conjunction with an increased number of irregular, jagged, vascular spaces lined by thin endothelial cells
- The vessels are mainly found in the upper part of the dermis
- In the tumoral stage, the spindle cells are arranged in interwoven fascicles with erythrocytes scattered in the interstices
- Plasma cells are present at all stages of the disease
- Nuclear atypia, pleomorphism and mitotic figures may be seen, but are usually not very prominent

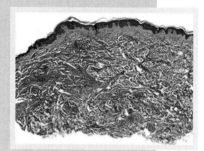

KAPOSI SARCOMA PATCH

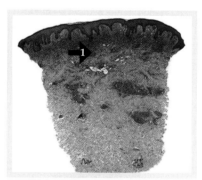

KAPOSI SARCOMA PLAQUE

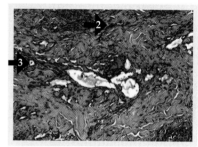

KAPOSI SARCOMA PLAQUE

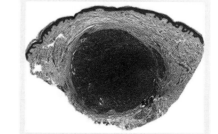

KAPOSI SARCOMA TUMOR

KAPOSI SARCOMA TUMOR

CLINICAL VARIANTS

- Classic
- Endemic
- Iatrogenic
- AIDS-associated

HISTOLOGICAL DIFFERENTIAL

1. Angiosarcoma:
- Irregular dissecting vascular spaces
- Atypical endothelial cells with nuclear pleomorphism and mitosis
- HHV-8 is negative
2. Benign lymphangioendothelioma:
- Multiple lesions present in a plate-like arrangement
- Negative HHV-8

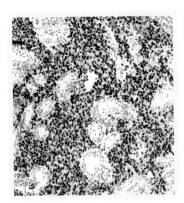

HHV-8 STAINING

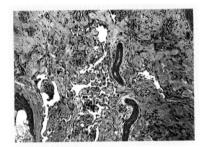

ANGIOSARCOMA

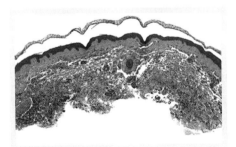

BENIGN LYMPHANGIOENDOTHELIOMA

PATHOPHYSIOLOGY

- They are the result of the complex interplay of HHV-8 with immunologic, genetic, and environmental factors

CLINICAL FEATURES

- There are three stages:
  o patch stage: brown-red macules or patches
  o plaque stage: brown-red and blue-violet Papules or plaques
  o tumor stage: violet nodules

SPECIAL STUDIES

- CD34+, CD31+, FLI1+, and HHV-8+

IMPORTANT THINGS TO KNOW

- The incidence of AIDS-related Kaposi sarcoma has decreased in the last few years

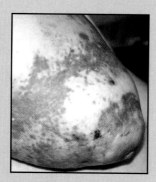

EPIDEMIOLOGY

- Usually affects the face or scalp in elderly patients, and it is more common in white people
- It also can affect the areas of chronic lymphedema, and chronic radiodermatitis

PATHOPHYSIOLOGY

- Arises from vascular endothelium. An alteration of the TP53/MDM2 pathway was documented in cases of angiosarcoma

CLINICAL FEATURES

- Clinically, angiosarcomas of the face appear as ill-defined bruise-like areas that simulate a hematoma
- More advanced lesions present as indurate plaques with raised, nodular, and occasionally ulcerated components accompanied by smaller satellite lesions in the vicinity

SPECIAL STUDIES

- D2-40+, CD31+, CD34+, HHV-8–

CLINICAL VARIANTS

- Idiopathic cutaneous angiosarcoma of the head and neck
- Lymphangiosarcoma arising in chronic lymphadematous limbs
- Postirradiation angiosarcoma

ANGIOSARCOMA

INTRODUCTION

Malignant neoplasm of endothelial cells with poor prognosis. There are three variants: angiosarcoma (AS) of the face and scalp; radiation-induced AS; and AS associated to chronic lymphedema.

HISTOLOGICAL FEATURES

1. Poorly circumscribed dermal tumor
2. Ectatic dissecting bizarre vessels
3. Atypical endothelial cells with nuclear pleomorphism and mitosis

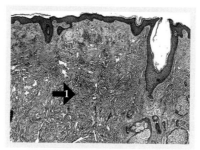

ANGIOSARCOMA   ANGIOSARCOMA

HISTOLOGICAL DIFFERENTIAL

1. Kaposi sarcoma:
- Spindle cell tumor with plasma cell
- Positive for HHV-8
- Endothelial cells are not atypical
2. Malignant melanoma:
- Positive for melanocytic markers such as S-100, HMB-45, Mart-1, and pan-melanoma
- Epidermal part of melanoma, if present, helps to differentiate

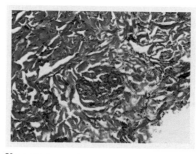

KAPOSI SARCOMA

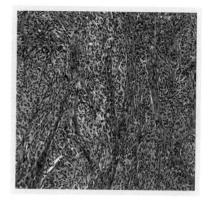

MALIGNANT MELANOMA

IMPORTANT THINGS TO KNOW

- Regardless of the variant of AS the histological features are similar

CUTANEOUS CYSTS

EPIDERMOID CYST (FOLLICULAR INFUNDIBULAR CYST/EPIDERMAL INCLUSION CYST)

INTRODUCTION

Epidermoid cyst is the most common cutaneous cyst. These can occurs anywhere, but are mostly seen on the face and upper trunk.

HISTOLOGICAL FEATURES

1. Cystic cavity filled with laminated keratin
2. Stratified squamous epithelium identical to the epidermis

Other features:
- Acute/chronic granulomatous inflammation (in case of rupture)

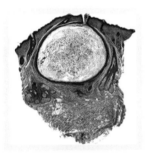

EPIDERMAL CYST

HISTOLOGICAL DIFFERENTIAL

Pilar cyst:
- Lack of granular layer
- Compact and homogenous contents (loose and flaky in epidermal cysts)
- Calcification may be present

Dilated pore of Winer:
- Communication with skin surface
- Epithelial lining is acanthotic
- Plate-like extensions and budding

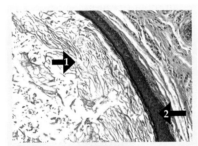

PILAR CYST

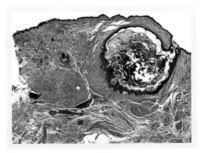

DILATED PORE OF WINER

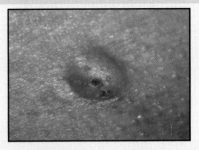

EPIDEMIOLOGY

- Young to middle-aged adults
- Seen on face, neck, upper trunk and scrotum

PATHOPHYSIOLOGY

- Derive mostly from follicular infundibulum
- May be primary but also can arise from traumatically implanted epithelium (true epidermal inclusion cysts) or disrupted follicular structures
- Multiple cysts can occur with Gardner syndrome and nevoid BCC syndrome
- Development of BCC or SCC within the cyst is very rare

CLINICAL FEATURES

- Well-demarcated, skin-colored or yellowish dermal nodules
- May have a visible punctum, representing the opening of the hair follicle from which the cyst arises
- Few millimeters to several centimeters in diameter
- Usually asymptomatic, but with pressure may release a creamy odorous content
- Rupture is accompanied by pain due to inflammation
- Tiny superficial cysts are known as milia
- Scrotal calcinosis is due to dystrophic calcification within multiple scrotal cysts

SPECIAL STUDIES

- None

CLINICAL VARIANTS

- None

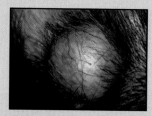

EPIDEMIOLOGY

- There is strong female preponderance

PATHOPHYSIOLOGY

- Pilar cysts arise from the isthmus of anagen hairs or from the sac surrounding catagen and telogen hairs, areas where the inner root sheath is lacking
- Proliferating trichilemmal cyst (PTC) or pilar tumor arises from irritation of a pre-existing pilar cyst. It is frequently described as a benign neoplasm, but potential for malignant transformation has been reported

CLINICAL FEATURES

- Pilar cysts occur predominantly on the scalp of elderly woman
- Usually solitary nodulocystic lesion, but can be multiple
- Size ranges from 1–10 cm in diameter
- Malignant PTC include: non-scalp location, size >5 cm and a history of a recent and rapid increase in size

SPECIAL STUDIES

- None

CLINICAL VARIANTS

- None

PILAR CYST (TRICHILEMMAL CYST)

INTRODUCTION

Benign epithelial lined cyst.

HISTOLOGICAL FEATURES

1. Lined by epithelium similar to the isthmic part of the hair follicle which is devoid of a granular layer (abrupt keratinization)
2. Peripheral palisading of nuclei
3. The cyst contents are made of a compact homogenous keratin
4. Calcification

Other features:
- Located in the middle to deep reticular dermis
- Absence of intercellular bridges between the keratinocytes
- Multinucleated keratinocytes (when ruptured)
- PTC consists of large, well-defined lobulated solid and cystic masses of proliferating keratinocytes with trichilemmal type of keratinization. The keratinocytes may exhibit cytological atypia and mitosis may be seen in the basal layer. Squamous eddies are seen
- Malignant PTC has infiltrative growth pattern, significant atypia and large number of mitotic figures

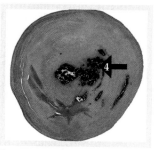

PILAR CYST

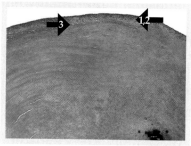

PILAR CYSTS

HISTOLOGICAL DIFFERENTIAL

1. Epidermal inclusion cyst:
- Lined by epithelium with prominent granular layer
- Stratum corneum laminated

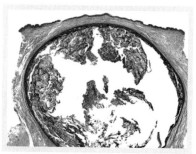

EPIDERMAL INCLUSION CYST

IMPORTANT THINGS TO KNOW

- Proliferating trichilemmal cyst is considered as a low-grade squamous cell carcinoma by some authors

Dermoid cyst

Introduction

Dermoid cysts are large lesions located in the dermis or subcutis and appear as discrete, subcutaneous nodules.

Histological features

1. Stratified squamous epithelium
2. Granular layer
3. Contains mature epidermal appendages connected to the wall

Other features:
- Hairs may project into the cyst wall
- Contains other normal structures like hair, eccrine glands, sebaceous lobules, apocrine glands, or smooth muscle

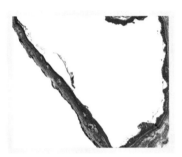 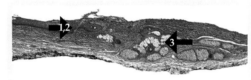

DERMOID CYST

Histological differential

1. Epidermoid cyst:
- Lack adnexal structures in wall
2. Steatocystoma:
- Wall of the cyst offers a crenulated appearance similar to the sebaceous duct
- Has eosinophilic cuticle on the luminal side of the epithelial lining
- Has sebaceous gland in cyst wall

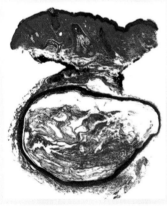 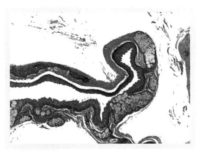

EPIDERMOID CYST   STEATOCYSTOMA

IMPORTANT THINGS TO KNOW

- Since neural heterotopias are included in the differential, imaging may be appropriate prior to rule out the possibility of connection with the CNS

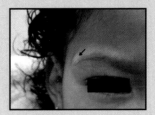

Epidemiology

- Present at birth, along an embryonic fusion plane
- May not be noticed until early childhood when they get inflamed, enlarged, or infected
- Rarely, they may go unnoticed until adulthood

Pathophysiology

- Congenital defect

Clinical features

- Well defined, rubbery, hard, raised, yellow-to-pink
- Fine hairs on surface may be seen
- 1–4 cm in diameter
- Most frequently seen around the eyes (especially lateral eyebrow) or midline of face. May be found on neck, sternum, sacrum, and scrotum
- May extend into the bone
- Lesions do not transilluminate

Special studies

- None

Clinical Variants

- None

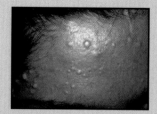

EPIDEMIOLOGY

- Usually appears at puberty

PATHOPHYSIOLOGY

- Autosomal dominant
- Mutations in the *KRT17* gene
- Possible androgenic influence
- Mechanism unknown:
  - o retention cysts versus
  - o dermoid cyst variant versus
  - o nevoid or hamartomatous condition of the pilar sebaceous duct zone

CLINICAL FEATURES

- Few millimeters to centimeters in diameter
- Most common on chest, axillae and groin
- Unusual variants include facial, acral, and a rare congenital linear form
- Persist indefinitely, but are asymptomatic

SPECIAL STUDIES

- None

CLINICAL VARIANTS

- Steatocystoma simplex
- Steatocystoma multiplex
- Facial
- Acral
- Congenital linear form

STEATOCYSTOMA

INTRODUCTION

Steatocystomas are dermal cysts that occur as single or multiple lesions (steatocystoma simplex versus multiplex) and drain oily fluid if punctured.

HISTOLOGICAL FEATURES

1. Dermal cyst lined by thin stratified squamous epithelium
2. No granular layer
3. Glassy, pink (eosinophilic) crenulated cuticle overlies the internal surface
4. Small sebaceous lobules in or adjacent to cyst wall

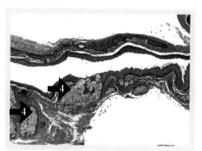
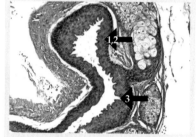

STEATOCYSTOMA   STEATOCYSTOMA

HISTOLOGICAL DIFFERENTIAL

1. Milia:
- Lacks the cuticle
- Lacks sebaceous glands in wall
2. Trichostasis spinulosa:
- Clinically unapparent
- Plugged follicle opens to surface with numerous vellus hairs
- Not a cyst

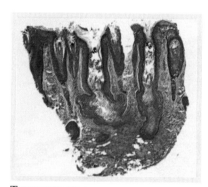

TRICHOSTASIS SPINULOSA

IMPORTANT THINGS TO KNOW

- Steatocystoma treated by excision/incision and removal of the cyst wall

BRONCHOGENIC CYST

INTRODUCTION

Bronchogenic cyst is the product of sequestered respiratory epithelium during embryologic development. They are located on the neck and within the thoracic cage surrounding the bronchial trees but may be localized to ectopic sites.

HISTOLOGICAL FEATURES

1. Lined by pseudostratified and ciliated columnar epithelium
2. Smooth muscle and mucous glands, and rarely cartilage, in cyst wall

Other features:
- Interspersed mucin-filled goblet cells within epithelium
- Metaplasia may lead to some areas of stratified squamous lining as well as ciliated columnar and goblet cells

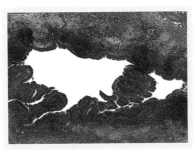

BRONCHOGENIC CYST

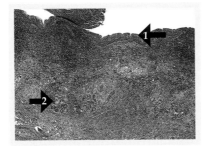

BRONCHOGENIC CYST

HISTOLOGICAL DIFFERENTIAL

1. Branchial cleft cyst:
- Presence of Lymphoid follicles
2. Cutaneous ciliated cyst:
- Clinical presentation and location

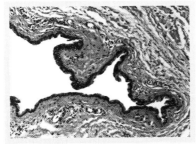

CUTANEOUS CILIATED CYST

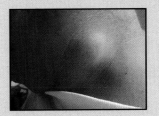

EPIDEMIOLOGY

- Usually present at birth
- Four times more common in males than females

PATHOPHYSIOLOGY

- Respiratory epithelium is sequestered during development of the embryonic tracheobronchial tree
- Migration of tissue to ectopic sites results in localization outside the developmental areas of the tracheal bronchial tree

CLINICAL FEATURES

- Solitary
- Commonly found in suprasternal notch
- Rarely seen on the anterior neck or chin, face, back, shoulder, or abdomen
- Located in subcutis and may be connected to epidermis via a fistulous tract
- Rarely present as a pedunculated growth

SPECIAL STUDIES

- None

IMPORTANT THINGS TO KNOW

- Malignant transformation is very rare

CLINICAL VARIANTS

- None

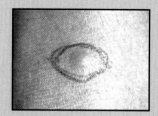

EPIDEMIOLOGY

- Young women; teen to young adults
- Rarely seen in men

PATHOPHYSIOLOGY

- Controversial
- Müllerian duct origin
- An alternative hypothesis seeks to explain the few cases in men and holds that eccrine glands undergo ciliated metaplasia

CLINICAL FEATURES

- Usually solitary, a few centimeters in diameter
- Lower extremities on young females, often on the sole but can be seen on buttocks
- Drain clear to amber fluid, if ruptured. Cyst usually appears empty due to rupture during biopsy

SPECIAL STUDIES

- None

CLINICAL VARIANTS

- None

CUTANEOUS CILIATED CYST

INTRODUCTION

Cutaneous ciliated cysts are uncommon and typically occur on the lower extremities of young women. This cyst is also known as cutaneous Müllerian cyst and cutaneous ciliated cystadenoma.

HISTOLOGICAL FEATURES

1. Unilocular or multiloculated
2. Located in subcutis or deep dermis
3. Simple cuboidal to columnar ciliated epithelium comprises the cyst wall
4. Papillary projections into the cyst lumen are common

Other features:
- May have areas of squamous metaplasia

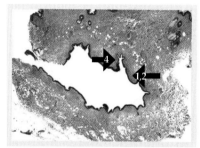

CUTANEOUS CILIATED CYST

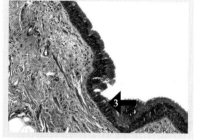

CUTANEOUS CILIATED CYST

HISTOLOGICAL DIFFERENTIAL

1. Bronchogenic cyst:
- Contains lymphoid tissue in wall
2. Thyroglossal duct cyst:
- Thyroid follicles in cyst wall

IMPORTANT THINGS TO KNOW

- Some suggest both cutaneous ciliated cyst and ciliated cyst of the vulva should be called cutaneous Müllerian cysts due to the same origin

MEDIAN RAPHE CYST

INTRODUCTION

Median raphe cyst (also known as apocrine cystadenoma of the penis) is a rare, small cyst occurring on the penis in young men.

HISTOLOGICAL FEATURES

1. Unilocular, irregularly shaped cystic spaces, not connecting to the overlying epithelium
2. Pseudostratified or stratified columnar epithelium, 1-4 cells layers thick

Other features:
- Mucin-containing cells
- Cyst may appear empty due to fluid leakage during biopsy
- Ciliated lining is very rare

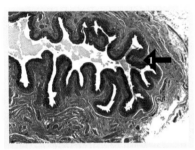

MEDIAN RAPHE CYST

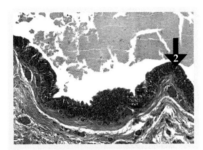

MEDIAN RAPHE CYST

HISTOLOGICAL DIFFERENTIAL

- Location and nature of lining make diagnosis obvious

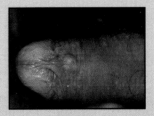

EPIDEMIOLOGY

- Young men

PATHOPHYSIOLOGY

- Develop due to aberrant urethral epithelium
- Caused by incomplete closure of urethral or genital folds or by outgrowths of embryologic epithelium occurring after primary closure of folds

CLINICAL FEATURES

- Solitary
- Usually a few millimeters in diameter, but may extend linearly over several centimeters
- Midline ventral aspect of the penis, on or near glans
- Do not connect to urethra

SPECIAL STUDIES

- None

IMPORTANT THINGS TO KNOW

- Treat by excision

CLINICAL VARIANTS

- None

CUTANEOUS METASTASES

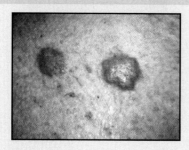

EPIDEMIOLOGY

- The incidence range from 1.2–4.4%. One study showed that the most common primary tumors in women were breast and in men were lung
- Cutaneous metastases are more likely to be seen in older individuals. In neonates they are usually derived from a neuroblastoma or rhabdomyosarcoma
- More than 60% are adenocarcinomas. About 15% are of squamous cell carcinomas. The rest are melanomas, undifferentiated neoplasms or others

PATHOPHYSIOLOGY

- The tumor cells may reach the skin by direct extension, by accidental implantation during a surgical procedure and by lymphatic and hematogenous spread

CLINICAL FEATURES

- Multiple, discrete, painless, freely movable nodules of sudden onset. They are usually 1–3 cm in diameter
- They vary in color from red to bluish purple to light brown or flesh color
- It tends to occur on the cutaneous surface near to the site of the primary tumor
- Approximately 5% of metastases involve the scalp
- Metastasis to the umbilicus is also quite common (Sister Mary Joseph nodule)

CUTANEOUS METASTASES

INTRODUCTION

Cutaneous metastasis may be the first indication of a visceral cancer. However, most metastases develop months or years after the primary malignancy has been diagnosed. Sometimes, cutaneous metastasis and the primary tumor are diagnosed simultaneously.

HISTOLOGICAL FEATURES

1. Metastases are centered on the dermis but they can extend into the subcutaneous tissue
2. The epidermis is usually spared, but it can be affected in some cases such as breast carcinoma (Paget's disease) or carcinomas of the bladder or colon (extramammary Paget's disease)

Other features:
- They may resemble the primary tumor. However, often it is necessary to perform special stains in order to determine the primary source of the neoplasm

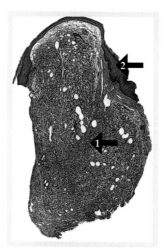

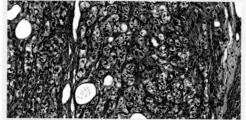

RENAL CELL CARCINOMA

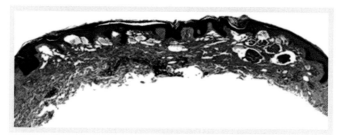

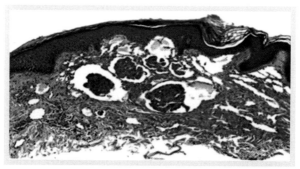

BREAST CARCINOMA

98

HISTOLOGICAL DIFFERENTIAL

The differential diagnosis depends on the primary source of the neoplasm. To cite a few examples:

- Clear cell hidradenoma: is the main differential diagnosis of renal cell carcinoma
- Endometriosis is the differential diagnosis of endometrial carcinoma and other adenocarcinomas.

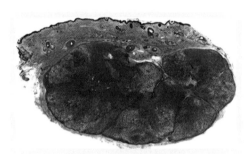

CLEAR CELL HIDRADENOMA

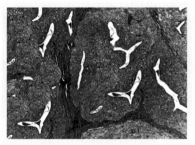

ENDOMETRIOSIS

IMPORTANT THINGS TO KNOW

- Metastatic melanoma can show epidermotropism
- The cells of metastatic lobular breast carcinoma have a linear array between collagen bundles

SPECIAL STUDIES

- Breast: CK7, GCDFP15, ER and PR are positive. CK20, CK5/6, S-100 &TTF-1 are negative
- Lung: CK7 and TTF-1 are positive. CK20,CK5/6, and S-100 are negative
- Thyroid: thyroglobulin, TTF-1 and CK7 are positive. CK20 is negative
- Kidney: RCC-Ma is positive. CK7 and CK20 are negative
- Colon: CK20 and CDx2 are positive. CK7 and TTF-1 are negative

CLINICAL VARIANTS

- None

CUTANEOUS INFILTRATES: NON-LYMPHOID

MAST CELL INFILTRATES

MASTOCYTOSIS

INTRODUCTION

Mastocytosis comprises a spectrum of related diseases in which there is an increase in mast cells in one or more organs. It is classified into cutaneous and systemic. Cutaneous mastocytosis includes: urticaria pigmentosa, solitary mastocytoma, diffuse cutaneous mastocytosis and telangectasia macularis eruptive perstans (TMEP). Systemic mastocytosis can be with or without cutaneous lesions.

HISTOLOGICAL FEATURES

1. The infiltrate is predominately in the upper third of the dermis
2. The number of mast cells depends on the clinical variant

Other features:
- Eosinophils variably present
- There are dense aggregates of mast cells in solitary mastocytoma and in some cases of urticaria pigmentosa. Loosely arranged mast cells are seen in diffuse cutaneous mastocytosis. In TMEP there may be only subtle alterations and only a few mast cells present

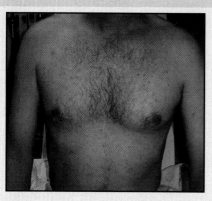

EPIDEMIOLOGY

- Although mastocytosis can occur at any age, usually the onset of mastocytosis is in the first 2 years of life (50% or more of the cases)
- Gender distribution is approximately equal

PATHOPHYSIOLOGY

- Two Kit mutations have been demonstrated which result in Kit autoactivation, and they are believed to be responsible for increased number of mast cells

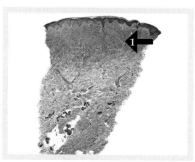

MASTOCYTOSIS

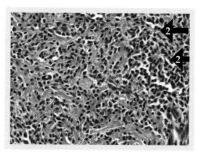

MASTOCYTOSIS

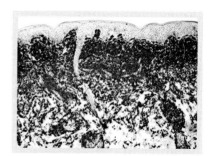

CD117 STAINING

HISTOLOGICAL DIFFERENTIAL

1. Melanocytic nevi:
- S-100 positive
2. Langerhans cell histiocytosis:
- CD1a and S-100 positive
- CD117 negative

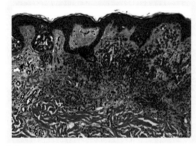

MELANOCYTIC NEVUS

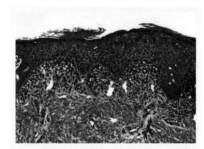

LANGERHANS CELL HISTIOCYTOSIS

IMPORTANT THINGS TO KNOW

- Subepidermal vesiculobullos changes may be seen with mast cell lesions of infancy

CLINICAL FEATURES

- Urticaria pigmentosa (the most common type) presents as a generalized eruption of multiple red macules mainly on the trunk. Less than 50% are pruritic
- Solitary mastocytoma may occur anywhere on the body with a predilection for the trunk
- Diffuse cutaneous mastocytosis is a rare variant begins in early infancy with thickening of the skin, pruritus and blistering are common
- TMEP is a rare adult form of mastocytosis. Telangectatic macules are found on the trunk
- More than 95% of adults but only a minority of children have systemic involvement

SPECIAL STUDIES

- Toluidine blue, Giemsa or chloroacetate esterase
- CD117 (C-kit) and mast cell tryptase are positive

CLINICAL VARIANTS

- Urticaria pigmentosa
- Solitary mastocytoma
- Diffuse cutaneous mastocytosis
- Telangectasia macularis eruptive perstans
- Systemic mastocytosis (can be with or without cutaneous lesions)

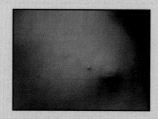

Epidemiology

- JXG affects mostly children with most of the cases diagnosed in the first year of life; however, similar lesions have been reported in adults

Pathophysiology

- The etiology of JXG is unknown

Clinical features

- Yellow-red to brown papules, most commonly seen on the head and neck, but can spread to the trunk and extremities
- A solitary lesion is seen in most of the cases, 10% of the cases present with multiple lesions

Special studies

- CD68+, factor XIII a+, S-100–, CD1a–

Juvenile xanthogranuloma

Introduction

Juvenile xanthogranuloma (JXG) is the most common non-Langerhans cell type of histiocytosis. Usually it is a self-limited disease.

Histological features

1. Diffuse collection of small monomorphous histiocytes are seen in the dermis, some of them with a foamy cytoplasm
2. Multitnucleated histiocytes (Touton cells)
3. Other inflammatory cells

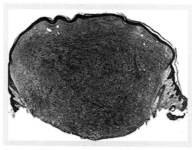
JUVENILE XANTHOGRANULOMA

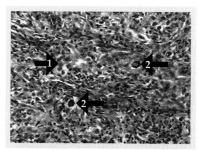
JUVENILE XANTHOGRANULOMA

Histological differential

1. Langerhans cell histiocytosis:
- Cells with eosinophilic cytoplasm and reniform (coffee bean) nuclei
- S-100+, CD1a+

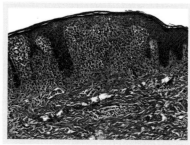
LANGERHANS CELL HISTIOCYTOSIS

Clinical Variants

- Benign cephalic histiocytosis
- Generalized eruptive histiocytosis
- Papular xanthogranuloma

Important Things To Know

- Early JXG consists of numerous histiocytes with abundant cytoplasm. Over time they become lipidized and Touton cells are identified

Xanthomas

Introduction

Xanthomas are group of infiltrates of foamy macrophages (histiocytes). They are often associated with hyperlipidemias (eruptive, tuberous, tendinous and xanthelasma) although others may be normolipemic (diffuse plane xanthoma, verruciform, papular and plexiform).

Histological features

1. Diffuse infiltrates of foamy histiocytes in the dermis
2. Variable numbers of other inflammatory cells

Other features:
- Eruptive xanthomas often have more inflammatory cells
- Multinucleated histiocytes are variably present in diffuse plane xanthomas and papular xanthomas
- In verruciform xanthomas, there is verrucous hyperplasia with parakeratosis and neutrophils
- In plexiform xanthomas, nodular collection of foamy macrophages merge with spindle-shaped cells arranged in large sweeping fascicles

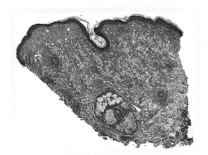

XANTHOMA

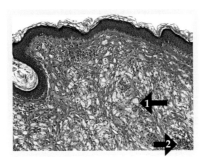

XANTHOMA

Histological differential

1. Langerhans cell histiocytosis:
- S-100+, CD1a+
2. Juvenile xanthogranuloma:
- Foamy histiocytes are less prominent

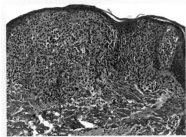

LANGERHANS CELL HISTIOCYTOSIS

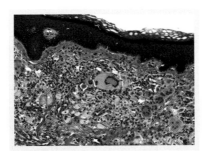

JUVENILE XANTHOGRANULOMA

IMPORTANT THINGS TO KNOW

- Xanthelasma is the most common form of xanthomas. Lipid levels are normal in around half of patients

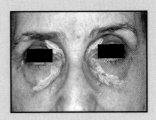

Epidemiology

- Papular xanthoma affects infants and children, whereas plexiform type affects middle-aged adult males. Other types have no age or sex predilection

Pathophysiology

- Xanthomas result when abnormalities in the transportation of lipids (e.g. cholesterol, triglycerides, and phospholipids) cause these lipids to be deposited in the skin and being ingested by tissue macrophages

Clinical features

- Yellow to brown papules, papules or plaques, those associated with hyperlipidemias have characteristic sites: elbows and knees (tuberous), Achilles tendon (tendinous), eyelid (xanthelasma), buttocks (eruptive)
- Diffuse planar xanthomas are distributed periorbitally, on the trunk and extremities. Verruciform is a solitary lesion in oral mucosa, papular xanthomas have a generalized distribution while plexiform xanthomas involve the lower extremities

Special studies

- CD68+, S-100–, CD1a–

Clinical Variants

- Tuberous xanthoma
- Planar xanthoma
- Tendinous xanthoma
- Eruptive xanthoma
- Plexiform xanthoma

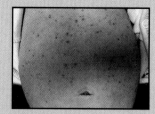

EPIDEMIOLOGY

- Although the disease can present at any age, most often it presents within the first few years of life with a slight male predominance

PATHOPHYSIOLOGY

- The etiology is unknown and there is considerable debate as to whether LCH is a reactive disorder or a neoplastic proliferation; however, the fact that the majority of cases studied have shown clonal proliferation of LC supports the latter hypothesis

CLINICAL FEATURES

- LCH can involve almost any organ system
- In children, LCH mostly present with multiorgan disease; however, adults more frequently have single system disease
- Bone is the most commonly affected organ. Mucocutaneous lesions are the second most common areas of involvement, often presenting as a papulosquamous eruption
- Prognosis is dependent upon the type and number of organs involved

SPECIAL STUDIES

- CD1a+, S-100+, langerin(CD207)+

CLINICAL VARIANTS

- Letterer-Siwe disease
- Eosinophilic granuloma
- Hand-Schuler-Christian disease

LANGERHANS CELL HISTIOCYTOSIS

INTRODUCTION

Langerhans cell histiocytosis (LCH) is a histioctytic disorder characterized by proliferation and accumulation of Langerhans cells (LC) into a variety of organs.

HISTOLOGICAL FEATURES

1. Clusters and sheets of large ovoid cells, immediately beneath the epidermis
2. Cells with abundant eosinophilic cytoplasm and a reniform and sometimes coffee bean shaped nucleus
3. Focally the cells invade the epidermis, forming small aggregates

Other features:
- Variable admixture of other inflammatory cells including: neutrophils, eosinophils, lymphocytes, and mast cells

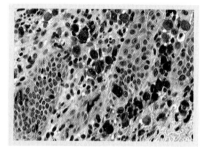

LANGERHANS CELL HISTIOCYTOSIS

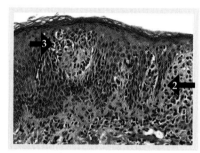

LANGERHANS CELL HISTIOCYTOSIS

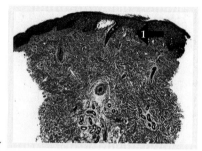

CD1A STAINING

HISTOLOGICAL DIFFERENTIAL

1. Juvenile xanthogranuloma:
- Multinucleated histiocytes (Touton cells)
- No involvement of the epidermis
- CD68+, S-100–, CD1a–
2. Xanthoma disseminatum:
- Mixture of histiocytes, foamy cells, multinucleated histiocytes
- CD68+, S-100–, CD1a–

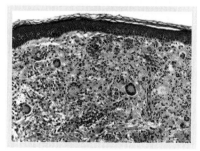

JUVENILE XANTHOGRANULOMA

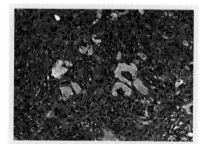

XANTHOMA DISSEMINATUM

IMPORTANT THINGS TO KNOW

- LC has Birbeck granules in cytoplasm detected by electron microscopy

Merkel cell carcinoma

Introduction

Merkel cell carcinoma (MCC) is a rare malignant primary cutaneous neoplasm with epithelial and neuroendocrine differentiation. The cell of origin remains unresolved.

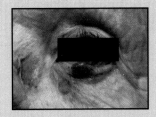

Histological features

Small, uniform round to oval blue cells with amphophilic sparse cytoplasm

Other features:
- Inconspicuous mitosis
- Apoptotic bodies are abundant
- The tumor has three different histological growth patterns, a sheet-like growth being the most common followed by the nested and trabecular types. It is centered on the dermis and frequently extends into the subcutaneous fat

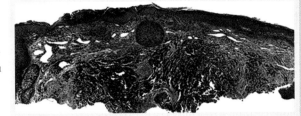

Merkel cell carcinoma

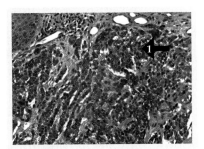

Merkel cell carcinoma

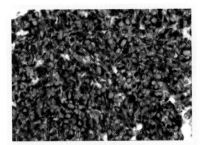

CK20 staining

Histological differential

1. Basal cell carcinoma:
- Peripheral palisading
- Myxoid stroma
- Chromogranin and synaptophysin are negative
2. Metastatic small cell carcinoma:
- TTF1 positive, MCPyV negative
3. Lymphoma:
- CD 45 positive, CK20 , chromogranin and synaptophysin are negative

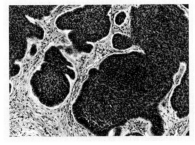

Basal cell carcinoma

Epidemiology

- The tumor most commonly affects white people
  - Male-to-female ratio is 2.3:1
  - It typically occurs on the sun-exposed skin of older adults
  - MCC is highly aggressive malignancy with more than 30% of patients dying within 5 years of diagnosis

Clinical features

- Solitary painless dome-shaped nodule or indurated plaque. Red, violaceous or skin-colored
- The most commonly affected sites are the head and neck and extremities.

Pathophysiology

- Immunosuppression state and UV irradiation are risk factors
- Merkel cell polyoma virus (MCPyV) DNA was demonstrated to be monoclonally integrated into the host genome in a majority of MCC

Special studies

- CK20 (paranuclear dots), AE1/AE3, CAM5.2, chromogranin, and synaptophysin are positive
- TTF1, CD45, S-100, and CK7 are negative. Minority of CK20–/CK7+ cases have been reported
- MCPyV positive in 80% of the cases

Important Things To Know

- Epidermis maybe involved in a pagetoid fashion
- Not infrequently, MCC occurs in intimate association with an in situ or invasive squamous cell carcinoma

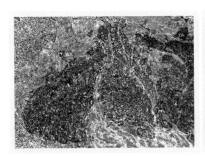

Metastatic small cell carcinoma

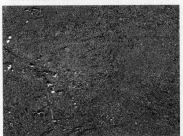

Lymphoma

Clinical Variants

- None

CUTANEOUS INFILTRATES: LYMPHOID AND LEUKEMIC

PSEUDOLYMPHOMAS

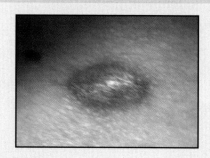

EPIDEMIOLOGY

- It affects all age groups. Drug-induced T-pseudolymphoma more frequently are seen in adults

PATHOPHYSIOLOGY

- Reactive polyclonal proliferation of T and B lymphocytes. It may be induced by microbial, physical or chemical agents

CLINICAL FEATURES

- Cutaneous lymphoid hyperplasia simulating B-cell lymphoma present as asymptomatic red brown nodules or papules. The most common sites of involvement are the face, chest and upper extremities
- Lymphomatoid drug reaction take the form of solitary plaques, nodules or multiple lesions with a wide spread distribution
- Pseudolymphomatous folliculitis present as solitary papule or nodule on the face

SPECIAL STUDIES

- B-cell markers CD20 and CD79 are present in some of the cells, while the T-cell marker CD3 is present in the majority of the cells. Polyclonal populations as demonstrated with the lambda and kappa light chains
- The germinal centers are highlighted by CD10 and BCL-6

CLINICAL VARIANTS

- None

CUTANEOUS PSEUDOLYMPHOMAS (LYMPHOID HYPERPLASIA)

INTRODUCTION

Cutaneous pseudolymphomas are benign lymphoid proliferations which simulate cutaneous lymphoma clinically and histopathologically.

HISTOLOGICAL FEATURES

1. In lymphoid hyperplasia simulating B-cell lymphoma there is dense diffuse cellular infiltrate, which is more often "top heavy".

Other Features:
- Lymphoid follicles are present in many but not all cases
- Tingible bodies inside macrophages are present
- Immunohistochemically, there is an admixture of B and T lymphocytes with a predominance of T-cell lymphocytes. No monocloanal populations are detected
- In lymphomatoid drug reaction the infiltrate may be band-like resembling mycosis fungoides or nodular
- Pseudolymphomatous folliculitis shows diffuse predominantly perifollicular infiltrate of lymphocytes with infiltration and destruction of follicular structures

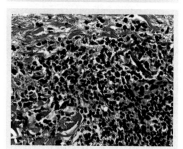

PSEUDOLYMPHOMA

HISTOLOGICAL DIFFERENTIAL

1. B-cell lymphoma:
- "Bottom-heavy" infiltrate
- Monoclonal populations are usually detected
- More than 50% of cells express B-cell markers

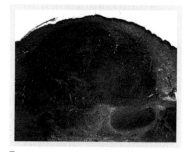

B-CELL LYMPHOMA

IMPORTANT THINGS TO KNOW

- Presence of monoclonal populations is not an absolute diagnostic criteria
- In reactions at site of vaccination, the subcutis is predominantly affected with little dermal involvement

T-CELL LYMPHOMAS

INTRODUCTION

Heterogeneous group of neoplasms, which show considerable variation in clinical presentation histopathology and prognosis. Mycosis fungoides (MF) is the most common T-cell lymphoma.

HISTOLOGICAL FEATURES

1. MF patch stage shows atypical lymphocytes in the epidermis (epidermotropism), typically confined to the basal layers either as single cells in a "string of beads" arrangement or as small groups of cells (Pautrier collections)
- The nuclei of the lymphocytes are cerebriform. Sparse infiltrate of lymphocytes spread along the papillary dermis
- Frequently there is papillary fibrosis
- In the plaque stage, the infiltrate is denser
- In the tumor stage the epidermotropism is uncommon and the entire dermis is often involved

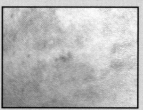

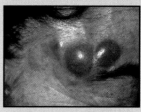

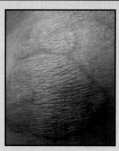

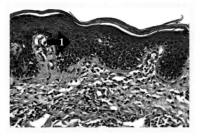

MF PATCH 2

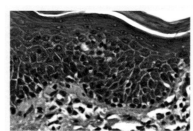

MF PATCH 3

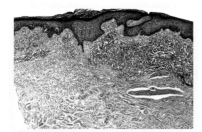

MF PLAQUE 2

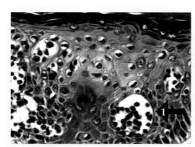

MF PAUTRIER COLLECTIONS

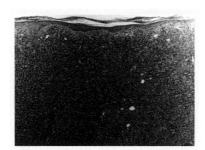

MF TUMORAL 2

EPIDEMIOLOGY

- MF usually arises in late adulthood with male predominance

PATHOPHYSIOLOGY

- Neoplastic cells in MF are mature T cells that express the cutaneous lymphocyte antigen (CLA), which enables them to specifically home into the skin.
- Etiology is unknown.

CLINICAL FEATURES

- MF is characterized by stepwise evolution with sequential appearance of patches, plaques and tumors. Pruritus is sometimes present. It has an indolent course

SPECIAL STUDIES

- MF: CD3+, CD4+, CD8–, CD30–, loss of CD5 and CD7

Histological differential

1. Spongiotic dermatitis:
- Areas of spongiosis predominate with a few lymphocytes present in the epidermis
- Lack of fibrosis of the papillary dermis
2. Drug reactions:
- May show similar features to MF, however, the lesions regress upon withdrawal of the offending drug

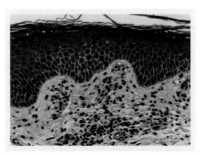

SPONGIOTIC DERMATITIS

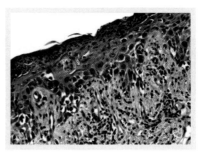

DRUG REACTION

Clinical Variants

- Granulomatous
- Hypopigmented
- Follicular
- Granulomatous slack skin syndrome
- Papular
- Solitary

Important Things To Know

- MF may show a protracted course and many times it takes several biopsies before a final diagnosis can be established

Primary cutaneous CD30+ T-cell lymphoproliferative disorders (lymphomatoid papulosis and anaplastic large cell lymphoma)

Introduction

Lymphomatoid papulosis (LyP) and anaplastic large cell lymphoma (ALCL) are chronic recurrent lymphoproliferative disease. The World Health Organization (WHO) classifies it within the spectrum of primary cutaneous CD30+ T-cell lymphoproliferative disorders with cutaneous anaplastic large cell lymphoma (C-ALCL)

Histological features

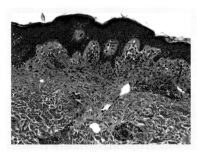

1. Diffuse infiltrates of atypical cells CD30+ present in the dermis
- Type A (Hodgkin-like) : wedge shape lesion with scattered, large , atypical CD4+/CD30+ cells in a mixed inflammatory background
- Type B (MF-like): small to medium atypical CD4+ cells which are often CD30 negative with scant inflammatory background and marked epidermotropism
- Type C (ALCL-like): sheets of large atypical CD4+/CD30+ cells
- Type D (Berti-like): sheets of medium and large sized atypical CD8+/CD30+ cells with scant or none inflammatory background and moderate epidermotropism by small and large cells
- Type E shows angiocentric infiltrates

LYMPHOMATOID PAPULOSIS

Histologic differential

1. Mycosis fungoides with large cell transformation:
- Patches or plaques clinically
- Band-like or diffuse infiltrate
- Moderate to marked epidermotropism
- Focal CD30 positivity
2. Arthropod bites:
- Diffuse infiltrate composed of lymphocytes and numerous eosinophils
- CD30–
3. Pityriasis lichenoides et varioliformis acuta (PLEVA):
- Areas of parakeratosis
- Dyskeratotic keratinocytes
- Absence of CD30+ cells

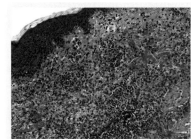

MYCOSIS FUNGOIDES

ARTHROPOD BITE

Important Things To Know

- Systemic and C-ALCL can be differentiated by the use of ALK stain, which is positive in the systemic variant and negative in C-ALCL

Epidemiology

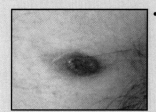

- LyP can affect patients of any age with peak incidence during the fifth decade. No major difference in gender distribution. Primary C-ALCL occurs in older adults and there is a male predominance. It is the second most common cutaneous T-cell lymphoma

Clinical features

- Recurrent and self-regressing red papules and nodules. May occur singly or in crops
- The size of the lesions is usually less than 1.5 cm or 2 cm, but more commonly they are smaller

Pathophysiology

- Whether LyP and C-ALCL represent indolent lymphomas. In both entities are characterized by t(2;5)(p23;q35)

Special studies

- Variable expression of CD4, CD8 and CD30 depends on the histologic type

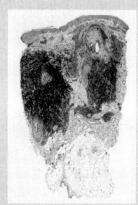

CD 30 STAINING

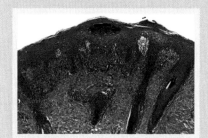

PITYRIASIS LICHENOIDES ET VARIOLIFORMIS ACUTA

Clinical Variants

- None

EPIDEMIOLOGY

- Primary cutaneous marginal zone lymphoma (PCMZL) and primary follicle center cell lymphoma occur in adults

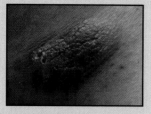

- PCMZL has a male predominance. DLBCL, leg type has a female predominance

PATHOPHYSIOLOGY

- PCMZL and DLBCL, leg type arise from post germinal center B-cells, primary cutaneous follicle center lymphoma arises from mature germinal center B-cells

CLINICAL FEATURES

- PCMZL occur mainly on the arms and trunk but other sides such as the head and neck may also be involved. The lesions are red to purple papules or nodules
- Lesions of follicle center lymphoma are usually single erythematous plaques or tumors; occur on the head and neck and trunk
- DLBCL, leg type occurs most frequently on the leg (72%) but can occur at other sites. The lesions present as rapidly growing erythematous tumors

SPECIAL STUDIES

- PCMZL: CD20+, CD79a+, bcl-2+, CD5–, CD10–, CD43–, cyclin D1–
- There is cytoplasmic immunoglobulin light chain restriction
- Follicle center lymphoma: CD20+, CD10+, bcl-6+, bcl-2 is negative
- DLBCL: CD20+, CD 79a+, bcl-6+, bcl-2+, MUM1/IRF4+

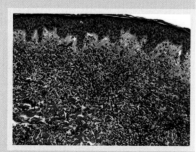

PSEUDOLYMPHOMA

CLINICAL VARIANTS

- None

B-CELL LYMPHOMA

INTRODUCTION

Cutaneous follicle center cell lymphoma and extranodal marginal zone B-cell lymphoma represent 90% of all forms of cutaneous B-cell lymphomas. Other cutaneous B-cell lymphomas are diffuse large B-cell lymphomas (DLBCL) of leg type, intravascular B-cell lymphoma and mantle cell lymphoma.

HISTOLOGICAL FEATURES

1. PCMZL shows a dermal cellular infiltrate that may extend into the subcutis but spares the epidermis
2. It has a nodular or diffuse pattern characterized by reactive lymphoid follicles surrounded by paler zone

Other features:

- They contain a mixed population of cells: small lymphocytes, centrocyte-like cells, monocytoid B-cells, lymphoplasmacytoid cells and plasma cells
- Follicular lymphoma may show follicular, follicular and diffuse, or diffuse patterns. Follicles are often variable in size and may fuse together. The follicle centers contain varying proportions of large and small centrocytes with cleaved nuclei and centroblasts with noncleaved nuclei and prominent nucleoli. Tangible body macrophages are absent
- DLBCL shows a diffuse infiltrate in the dermis and subcutis of large lymphocytes with features of centroblasts and immunoblasts, mitotic figures are common
- Other types of DLBCL in the skin are intravascular large B-cell lymphoma, plasmablastic lymphoma, DLBCL leg type

HISTOLOGICAL DIFFERENTIAL

1. Pseudolymphoma:
- Usually top heavy versus bottom heavy in lymphomas
- Lymphoid follicles have obvious tangible body macrophages
- Plasma cells in pseudolymphoma are polyclonal and monoclonal in PCMZL

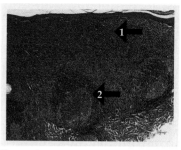

PRIMARY CUTANEOUS MARGINAL ZONE LYMPHOMA (PCMZL)

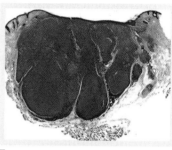

FOLLICULAR LYMPHOMA

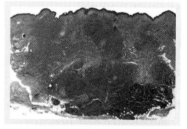

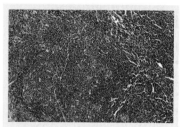

DIFFUSE LARGE B-CELL LYMPHOMAS (DLBCL)

IMPORTANT THINGS TO KNOW

- Plasmacytoid cells are a clue to PCMZL
- Unlike follicular lymphoma of lymph nodes, the t(14:18) is not found in primary cutaneous cases

LEUKEMIA CUTIS

INTRODUCTION

Cutaneous infiltrate of leukemic cells of acute or chronic myeloid leukemias (AML and CML, respectively), lymphoid leukemias, and in the setting of myelodysplastic and myeloproliferative syndromes.

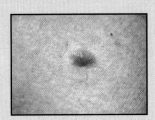

HISTOLOGICAL FEATURES

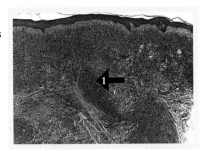

1. Sheets of atypical cells involve the dermis and subcutis

Other features:
- There may be destruction of the appendages by periappendageal infiltrate
- Sometimes there is percolation between collagen bundles in an "Indian file pattern"
- In CML the infiltrate is more pleomorphic with immature and mature granulocytes
- In PBLA the infiltrate consist of medium-sized lymphoid cells with round or convoluted nuclei, inconspicuous nucleoli and scant basophilic cytoplasm
- Mitosis and apoptotic bodies are often seen
- CLL/SLL: diffuse or nodular infiltrate of small mature lymphocytes

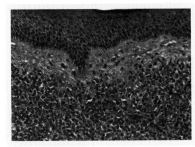

LEUKEMIA CUTIS

HISTOLOGICAL DIFFERENTIAL

1. T-cell lymphomas:
- T-cell markers are positive CD3, CD4 or CD8
2. Merkel cell carcinoma:
- Negative lymphoid markers
- Positive for CD20 and polyoma virus

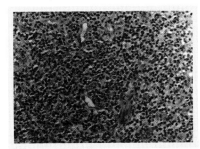

T-CELL LYMPHOMAS

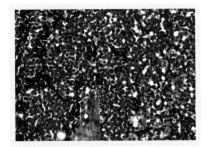

MERKEL CELL CARCINOMA

IMPORTANT THINGS TO KNOW

- Leukemia in biopsies show superficial and deep infiltrate with perieccrine and perivascular distribution. "Indian file pattern" is a clue in myeloid leukemia

EPIDEMIOLOGY

- Cutaneous involvement in AML is in the range of 2–20%, particularly M4 and M5, and in CML, 0–4%. Males and females are equally affected, mostly adults
- Precursor B-cell leukemia/lymphoma (PBLA) is more common in the skin than those of precursor T-cell origin (PTLA). Children are mostly affected. Skin is involved in 2% of chronic lymphocytic leukemia/small lymphocytic lymphoma (CLL/SLL)

PATHOPHYSIOLOGY

- Leukemia arises from hematopoietic stem cells in the bone marrow. Down syndrome and Fanconi anemia predispose to AML. CML associated with t(9:22)
- CLL/SLL and PBLA are of B-cell origin

CLINICAL FEATURES

- Myeloid leukemia present as single or multiple macules, papules, nodules or plaques with red/brown color in no particular distribution. Gum infiltration is common in M5
- PBLA and PTLA: erythematous papules or nodules mostly on the head and neck

SPECIAL STUDIES

- Myeloid leukemia: myeloperoxidase, CD43+ CD11+, lysozyme+. CD3–, CD20–
- PBLA: CD45+, CD79a+, CD10+, CD99+, Tdt+, CD20+ less commonly
- CLL/SLL: CD45+, CD20+, CD5+, CD23+, CD10–, cyclinD1–

CLINICAL VARIANTS

- None

REFERENCES

1 TUMORS OF THE EPIDERMIS

EPIDERMAL NEVUS

Adams B, Mutasim D: Adult onset verrucous epidermal nevus. *J Am Acad Dermatol* 1999;41:824–6.

Alsaleh QA, Nanda A, Hassab-el-Naby HM, Sakr MF. Familial inflammatory linear verrucous epidermal nevus (ILVEN). *Int J Dermatol* 1994;33:52–4.

Requena L, Requena C, Cockerell CJ. Benign epidermal tumors and proliferations. In: Bolognia J, Jorizzo J, Schaffer J (eds) *Dermatology* 3e. St Louis: Elsevier Saunders 2012:1809–10.

Solomon LM, Esterly NB. Epidermal and other congenital organoid nevi. *Curr Probl Pediatr* 1975;6(1):1–56.

Vidaurri-de la Cruz H1, Tamayo-Sánchez L, Durán-McKinster C, de la Luz Orozco-Covarrubias M, Ruiz-Maldonado R. Epidermal nevus syndromes: Clinical findings in 35 patients. *Pediatr Dermatol* 2004;21:432–9.

Weedon D. *Weedon's Skin Pathology* 3e. Edinburgh: Elsevier/Churchill Livingstone; 2010: 668-9.

CLEAR CELL ACANTHOMA

Barnhill, RL. Tumors of the epidermis. In *Dermatopathology*. New York: McGraw-Hill Medical; 2010:568–69.

Elston D, Ferringer T. *Requisites in Dermatology: Dermatopathology,* London: Elsevier/Saunders 2009: 41,78.

Murphy R, Kesseler ME, Slater DM. Giant cell acanthoma. *Br J Dermatol* 2000;143:1114-1115.

Requena L, Requena C, Cockerell CJ. Benign epidermal tumors and proliferations. In: Bolognia J, Jorizzo J, Schaffer J (eds) *Dermatology* 3e. St Louis: Elsevier Saunders 2012:1809-10.

Thomas VD, Swanson NA, Lee KK. Benign epithelial tumors, hamartomas, and hyperplasias. In Wolff K, Goldsmith LA, Katz SI, Gilchrest B, Paller AS, Leffell DJ (eds) *Fitzpatrick's Dermatology in General Medicine*, 7e. New York: McGraw-Hill; 2012.

Zedek CD, Langel DJ, White WL. Clear cell acanthoma acanthosis: a psoriasiform reaction pattern lacking tricholemmal differentation. *Am J Dermatopathol.* 2007;29:378–84

VIRAL WARTS

Barnhill RL, Crowson AN, Magro CM, Piepkorn MW (eds). *Dermatopathology* 3e. New York: McGraw-Hill; 2010:507-9.

Weedon D. *Weedon's Skin Pathology* 3e. Edinburgh: Churchill Livingstone; 2010: 619-24.

TRICHOLEMMOMA (TRICHILEMMOMA)

Ackerman AB, Reddy VB, Soyer HP. Neoplasms with follicular differentiation 2e. New York: Ardor Scribendi; 2001: 1109.

Brownstein, M.H., Trichilemmoma. Benign follicular tumor or viral wart? *Am J Dermatopathol* 1980;2:229–31.

Elston D, Ferringer T. Requisites in Dermatology: Dermatopathology, London: Elsevier/Saunders 2009: 78.

Hunt SJ, Kilzer B, Santa Cruz DJ. Desmoplastic trichilemmoma: histologic variant resembling invasive carcinoma. *J Cutan Pathol* 1990;17:45–52.

Illueca C, Monteagudo C, Revert A, et al. Diagnostic value of CD34 immunostaining in desmoplastic trichilemmoma. *J Cutan Pathol* 1998;25:435–439.

Leonardi CL, Zhu WY, Kinsey WH, Penneys NS. Trichilemmomas are not associated with human papillomavirus DNA. *J Cutan Pathol* 1991;18:193–7.

McCalmont TH. Adnexal neoplasms. In Bolognia J, Jorizzo J, Schaffer J (eds) *Dermatology* 3e. St Louis: Elsevier/Saunders 2012:1836-7.

INVERTED FOLLICULAR KERATOSIS

Azzopardi, J, Laurini, R. Inverted Follicular Keratosis. *J Clin Pathol* 1975;28:465–71.

Requena L, Requena C, Cockerell CJ. Benign epidermal tumors and proliferations. In: Bolognia J, Jorizzo J, Schaffer J (eds) *Dermatology* 3e. St Louis: Elsevier Saunders 2012:1806.

SOLAR LENTIGO

Barnhill, RL. Tumors of the epidermis. In *Dermatopathology*. New York: McGraw-Hill Medical; 2010: 615–6.

Weedon D. *Weedon's Skin Pathology* 3e. Edinburgh: Churchill Livingstone; 2010: 619–24.

SEBORRHEIC KERATOSIS

Mandinova A, Kolev V, Neel V, et al: A positive FGFR3/FOXN1 feedback loop underlies benign skin keratosis versus squamous cell carcinoma formation in humans. *J Clin Invest* 2009;119:3127–37.

McKee PH, Calonje E, Granter SR. Tumors of surface epithelium. In *Pathology of the Skin with Clinical Correlations* 3e. Edinburgh:Elsevier/Mosby 2005:1158–63.

Requena L, Requena C, Cockerell CJ. Benign epidermal tumors and proliferations. In: Bolognia J, Jorizzo J, Schaffer J (eds) *Dermatology* 3e. St Louis: Elsevier Saunders 2012:1795-8

WARTY DYSKERATOMA

Barnhill, RL. Tumors of the epidermis. In *Dermatopathology*. New York: McGraw-Hill Medical; 2010: 563–4.

LeBoit PE, Burg G, Weedon D, Sarasin A. *Pathology and Genetics of Skin Tumours*. Lyon: IARC Press; 2006.

BASAL CELL CARCINOMA

Barnhill RL, Crowson AN (eds). *Textbook of Dermatopathology* 2e. New York: McGraw-Hill 2004: 599–608.

Rapini R. *Practical Dermatopathology*. London:Elsevier/Mosby; 2005: 249–52.

Soyer PH, Rigel DS, Wurm EMT. Actinic keratosis, basal cell carcinoma and squamous cell carcinoma. In: Bolognia J, Jorizzo J, Schaffer J (eds) *Dermatology* 3e. St Louis: Elsevier Saunders 2012:1784-88.

Wolff K, Johnson RA, Suurmond D. *Fitzpatrick's Color Atlas and Synopsis of Clinical Dermatology* 5e. New York: McGraw-Hill; 2005: 282–91.

BOWEN'S DISEASE

LeBoit PE, Burg G, Weedon D, Sarasain A (eds). *World Health Orgnization Classification of Tumors. Pathology and Genatics of Skin Tumors*. Lyon: IARC Press; 2006; 29–31.

Weedon D. *Weedon's Skin Pathology* 3e. Edinburgh: Churchill Livingstone; 2010:679–81.

KERATOACANTHOMA

Barnhill RL, Crowson AN, Magro CM, Piepkorn MW (eds). Dermatopathology 3e. New York: McGraw-Hill;2010: 576–8.

Weedon D. *Weedon's Skin Pathology* 3e. Edinburgh: Churchill Livingstone; 2010:679–81.702-4

SQUAMOUS CELL CARCINOMA

Arbiser JL, Fan CY, Su X, et al. Involvement of p53 and p16 tumor suppressor genes in recessive dystrophic epidermolysis bullosa-associated squamous cell carcinoma. *J Invest Dermatol* 2004;123:788–90.

Boyd AS. Tumors of the epidermis. In Barnhill RL, Crowson AN (eds) *Textbook of Dermatopathology* 2e. New York: McGraw-Hill; 2004: 612–5.

Brown VL, Harwood CA, Crook T, Cronin JG, Kelsell DP, Proby CM. p16INK4a and p14ARF tumor suppressor genes are commonly inactivated in cutaneous squamous cell carcinoma. *J Invest Dermatol* 2004;122:1284–92.

de Gruijl FR, Rebel H. Early events in UV carcinogenesis: DNA damage, target cells and mutant p53 foci. *Photochem Photobiol* 2008;84:382–7.

Johnson TM, Rowe DE, Nelson BR, Swanson NA. Squamous cell carcinoma of the skin (excluding lip and oral mucosa). *J Am Acad Dermatol* 1992;26:467–84.

LeBoit, PE. Can we understand keratoacanthoma? *Am Dermatopathol* 2002;24:166–8.

Ziegler A, Jonason AS, Leffell DJ, et al. Sunburn and p53 in the onset of skin cancer. *Nature* 1994;372:773–6.

2 MELANOCYTIC NEOPLASMS

LENTIGO SIMPLEX (JUVENILE LENTIGO)

Elder D, Elenitsas R, Jaworsky C, Johnson R Jr. *Lever's Histopathology of the Skin* 10e. Philadelphia: Lippincott-Raven; 2008: 708–12.

Rabinovitz HS, Barnhill RL. Benign melanocytic neoplasms. In Bolognia J, Jorizzo J, Schaffer J (eds). *Dermatology* 3e. St Louis: Elsevier/Saunders; 2012: 1855–8.

Wolff K, Goldsmith LA, Katz SI, Gilchrest BA, Paller AS, Leffell DJ, eds. *Fitzpatrick's Dermatology In General Medicine* 7e. New York: McGraw-Hill; 2008: 1117–9.

MELANOCYTIC NEVI

Elder D, Elenitsas R, Jaworsky C, Johnson R Jr. *Lever's Histopathology of the Skin* 10e. Philadelphia: Lippincott-Raven; 2008: 711–4.

Massi G, LeBoit PE, Pasquini P. *Histological Diagnosis of Nevi and Melanoma*. Darmstadt: Steinkopff-Verlag Darmstadt; 2004: 49.

Penneys NS, Mogollon R, Kowalczyk A, et al. A survey of cutaneous neural lesions for the presence of myelin basic protein. An immunohistochemical study. *Arch Dermatol* 1984;120:210–3.

Rabinovitz HS, Barnhill RL. Benign melanocytic neoplasms. In Bolognia J, Jorizzo J, Schaffer J (eds). *Dermatology* 3e. St Louis: Elsevier/Saunders; 2012: 1861-3

Wolff K, Goldsmith LA, Katz SI, Gilchrest BA, Paller AS, Leffell DJ, eds. *Fitzpatrick's Dermatology In General Medicine* 7e. New York: McGraw-Hill; 2008: 178–81.

HALO NEVUS (SUTTON'S NEVUS)

Moschella SL, Hurley HJ. *Dermatology* 3e. Philadelphia: Saunders; 1992: 1751–75.

Rabinovitz HS, Barnhill RL. Benign melanocytic neoplasms. In Bolognia J, Jorizzo J, Schaffer J (eds). *Dermatology* 3e. St Louis: Elsevier/Saunders; 2012: 1875–6.

SPITZ NEVUS

Elder D, Elenitsas R, Jaworsky C, Johnson R Jr. Lever's Histopathology of the Skin 10e. Philadelphia: Lippincott-Raven; 2008: 718–24.

Fass J, Grimwood RE, Kraus E, et al. Adult onset of eruptive widespread Spitz's nevi. *J Am Acad Dermatol* 2002;46:S142–3.

Hulshof MM, Van Haeringen A, Gruis NA, et al. Multiple agminate Spitz naevi. *Melanoma Res* 1998;8:156–60.

Mencía-Gutiérrez E, Gutiérrez-Diaz E, Madero-García S. Juvenile xanthogranuloma of the orbit in an adult. *Ophthalmologica* 2000;214:437–0.

Paniago-Pereira C, Maize JC, Ackerman AB. Nevus of large spindle and /or epithelioid cells (Spitz's nevus). *Arch Dermatol* 1978;114:1811–23.

Rabinovitz HS, Barnhill RL. Benign melanocytic neoplasms. In Bolognia J, Jorizzo J, Schaffer J (eds). *Dermatology* 3e. St Louis: Elsevier/Saunders; 2012: 1864–7.

Weedon D, Little JH. Spindle and epithelioid cell nevi in children and adults. A review of 211 cases of the Spitz nevus. *Cancer* 1977;40:217–25.

Wolff K, Johnson RA. *Fitzpatrick's Color Atlas and Synopsis of Clinical Dermatology* 6e. New York: McGraw-Hill; 2009: 188.

Blue nevus

McKee PH, Calonje E, Granter SR. Melanocytic nevi. In: *Pathology of the Skin with Clinical Correlations* 3e. Edinburgh: Elsevier/Mosby 2005; 1299–1308.

Murali R, McCarthy SW, Scolyer RA: Blue nevi and related lesions: a review highlighting atypical and newly described variants, distinguishing features and diagnostic pitfalls. *Adv Anat Pathol* 2009;16:365–82.

Rabinovitz HS, Barnhill RL. Benign melanocytic neoplasms. In Bolognia J, Jorizzo J, Schaffer J (eds). *Dermatology* 3e. St Louis: Elsevier/Saunders; 2012: 1860–1.

Weedon D. *Weedon's Skin Pathology* 3e. Edinburgh: Elsevier/Churchill Livingstone; 2010: 728–9.

Malignant melanomas and variants

Elder D, Elenitsas R, Jaworsky C, Johnson R Jr. *Lever's Histopathology of the Skin* 10e. Philadelphia: Lippincott-Raven; 2008: 738–75.

Garbe C, Bauer J. Melanoma. In Bolognia J, Jorizzo J, Schaffer J (eds). *Dermatology* 3e. St Louis: Elsevier/Saunders; 2012: 1885–1910.

Wolff K, Goldsmith LA, Katz SI, Gilchrest BA, Paller AS, Leffell DJ, eds. *Fitzpatrick's Dermatology In General Medicine* 7e. New York: McGraw-Hill; 2008: 1134–57.

3 Tumors of Cutaneous Appendages

Trichoepithelioma

Barnhill RL, Crowson AN (eds). *Textbook of Dermato*pathology 2e. New York: McGraw-Hill 2004: 722–24.

Elston D, Ferringer T. *Requisites in Dermatology: Dermatopathology*, London: Elsevier/Saunders 2009: 71–2.

Rapini R. *Practical Dermatopathology*. London: Elsevier/Mosby; 2005: 286-304

Soyer PH, Rigel DS, Wurm EMT. Actinic keratosis, basal cell carcinoma and squamous cell carcinoma. In: Bolognia J, Jorizzo J, Schaffer J (eds) *Dermatology* 3e. St Louis: Elsevier Saunders 2012: 1784–88, 1835.

Weedon D. *Weedon's Skin Pathology* 3e. Edinburgh: Elsevier/Churchill Livingstone; 2010: 760–2.

Wolff K, Johnson RA, Suurmond D. Fitzpatrick's Color *Atlas and Synopsis of Clinical Dermatology* 5e. New York: McGraw-Hill; 2005: 210.

Trichoblastoma

Barnhill, R, Crowson AN, Magro CM, Piepkorn MW. *Dermatopathology*. New York: McGraw-Hill; 2010: 709–10.

Johnston RB. *Weedon's Skin Pathology Essentials*. Edinburgh: Elsevier/Churchill Livingstone; 2012: 567.

Trichofolliculoma

Elston D, Ferringer T. *Requisites in Dermatology: Dermatopathology*. London: Elsevier/Saunders 2009: 76–8.

McCalmont T. Adnexal neoplasms. In Bolognia J, Jorizzo J, Schaffer J (eds) *Dermatology* 3e. Philadelphia: Elsevier/Saunders; 2012: 1829–30.

Weedon D. *Weedon's Skin Pathology* 3e. Edinburgh: Elsevier/Churchill Livingstone; 2010: 758–9.

Pilar sheath acanthoma

Barnhill, R, Crowson AN, Magro CM, Piepkorn MW. Pilar sheath acanthoma. In *Dermatopathology*. New York: McGraw-Hill; 2010: 697–8.

Mehregan AH, Brownstein MH. Pilar sheath acanthoma. *Arch Dermatol* 1978:114:1495–97.

Tumor of the follicular infundibulum

Barnhill, R, Crowson AN, Magro CM, Piepkorn MW. Tumor of the follicular infundibulum. In *Dermatopathology*. New York: McGraw-Hill; 2010: 697,700.

McCalmont T. Adnexal neoplasms. In Bolognia J, Jorizzo J, Schaffer J (eds) *Dermatology* 3e. Philadelphia: Elsevier/Saunders; 2012: 1837–8.

Sebaceous hyperplasia

Boschnakow A, May T, Assaf C, Tebbe B, Zouboulis C. Ciclosporin A-induced sebaceous gland hyperplasia. *Br J Dermatol* 2003;149:198–200.

Bryden AM, Dawe RS, Fleming C. Dermatoscopic features of benign sebaceous proliferation. *Clin Exp Dermatol* 2004;29:676–7.

Deplewski D, Rosenfield RL. Role of hormones in pilosebaceous unit development. *Endocr Rev* 2000;21:363-92.

Elder D, Elenitsas R, Ragsdale BD. Tumors of the epidermal appendages. In: Elder D, Elenitas R, Jaworsky C, Johnson B (eds) *Lever's Histopathology of the Skin* 8e. Philadelphia: Lippincott-Raven; 1997: 719–46.

McCalmont T. Adnexal neoplasms. In Bolognia J, Jorizzo J, Schaffer J (eds) *Dermatology* 3e. Philadelphia: Elsevier/Saunders; 2012: 1839.

Zaballos P, Ara M, Puig S, Malvehy J. Dermoscopy of sebaceous hyperplasia. *Arch Dermatol* 2005;141:808.

Sebaceoma

McCalmont T. Adnexal neoplasms. In Bolognia J, Jorizzo J, Schaffer J (eds) *Dermatology* 3e. Philadelphia: Elsevier/Saunders; 2012: 1839–40.

Steffen C, Ackerman AB. *Neoplasms with Sebaceous Differentiation*. Philadelphia: Lea & Febiger; 1994.

Troy JL, Ackerman AB. Sebaceoma: a distinctive benign neoplasm of adnexal epithelium differentiating toward sebaceous cells. *Am J Dermatopathol* 1984;6:7.

Weedon D. Weedon's Skin Pathology 3e. Edinburgh: Elsevier/Churchill Livingstone; 2010: 776.

Sebaceous adenoma

McCalmont T. Adnexal neoplasms. In Bolognia J, Jorizzo J, Schaffer J (eds) *Dermatology* 3e. Philadelphia: Elsevier/Saunders; 2012: 1839–40.

Suspiro A, Fidalgo P, Cravo M, Albuquerque C, Ramalho E, Leitão CN, et al. The Muir-Torre syndrome: a rare variant of hereditary nonpolyposis colorectal cancer associated with hMSH2 mutation. *Am J Gastroenterol* 1998;93:1572–4.

Troy JL, Ackerman AB. Sebaceoma. A distinctive benign neoplasm of adnexal epithelium differentiating toward sebaceous cells. *Am J Dermatopathol* 1984;6:7–13.

Wick MR, Swanson PE, Barnhill RL. Sebaceous and pilar tumors. In Barnhill, RL, Crowson, AN (eds) *Textbook of Dermatopathology*. New York: McGraw-Hill; 2004: 710–1.

SEBACEOUS CARCINOMA

Buitrago W Joseph AK. Sebaceous carcinoma: the great masquerader. Dermatol Ther 2008; 21:459–66.

McCalmont T. Adnexal neoplasms. In Bolognia J, Jorizzo J, Schaffer J (eds) *Dermatology* 3e. Philadelphia: Elsevier/ Saunders; 2012: 1840.

Weedon D. *Weedon's Skin Pathology* 3e. Edinburgh: Elsevier/ Churchill Livingstone; 2010: 777–8.

APOCRINE ADENOMA

Barnhill R, Crowson AN, Magro CM, Piepkorn MW. *Dermatopathology*. New York: McGraw-Hill; 2010. 731,735.

Johnston RB. *Weedon's Skin Pathology Essentials*. Edinburgh: Elsevier/Churchill Livingstone; 2012: 591.

McCalmont T. Adnexal neoplasms. In Bolognia J, Jorizzo J, Schaffer J (eds) *Dermatology* 3e. Philadelphia: Elsevier/ Saunders; 2012: 1843–4.

Wolff K, Johnson RA, Fitzpatrick TB. Appendage tumors with apocrine differentiation. In: *Fitzpatrick's Color Atlas and Synopsis of Clinical Dermatology*. New York: McGraw-Hill; 2009: 1071–2.

SYRINGOCYSTADENOMA PAPILLIFERUM

Barnhill R, Crowson AN, Magro CM, Piepkorn MW. Syringocystadenoma papilliferum. In *Dermatopathology*. New York: McGraw-Hill; 2010: 734–5

Bolognia, J, Jorizzo JL, Rapini RP (eds). Nevus sebaceus. In *Dermatology* 2e. St Louis: Elsevier/Mosby; 2008. 1695–96.

Ghosh SK, Bandyopadhyay D, Chatterjee G, Bar C. Syringocystadenoma papilliferum: An unusual presentation. *Pediatr Dermatol* 2009;26:758–9.

Johnston RB. *Weedon's Skin Pathology Essentials*. Edinburgh: Elsevier/Churchill Livingstone; 2012: 590.

Leeborg N, Thompson M, Rossmiller S, Gross N, White C, Gatter K. Diagnostic pitfalls in syringocystadenocarcinoma papilliferum: Case report and review of the literature. *Arch Pathol Lab Med* 2010;134:1205–9

McCalmont T. Adnexal neoplasms. In Bolognia J, Jorizzo J, Schaffer J (eds) *Dermatology* 3e. Philadelphia: Elsevier/ Saunders; 2012: 1843-4.

HIDRADENOMA

Barnhill R, Crowson AN, Magro CM, Piepkorn MW. In *Dermatopathology*. New York: McGraw-Hill; 2010: 731–3.

Johnston RB. *Weedon's Skin Pathology Essentials*. Edinburgh: Elsevier/Churchill Livingstone; 2012: 592,605.

McCalmont T. Adnexal neoplasms. In Bolognia J, Jorizzo J, Schaffer J (eds) *Dermatology* 3e. Philadelphia: Elsevier/ Saunders; 2012: 1842–3

CYLINDROMA

Barnhill R, Crowson AN, Magro CM, Piepkorn MW. In *Dermatopathology*. New York: McGraw-Hill; 2010: 725

Breathnach S. Drug Reactions. In Burns T, Breathnach S, Cox N, Griffiths C (eds) *Rook's Textbook of Dermatology* 7e. Oxford: Blackwell Publishing; 2004.

Johnston RB. *Weedon's Skin Pathology Essentials*. Edinburgh: Elsevier/Churchill Livingstone; 2012: 594

Lee MW, Kelly JW. Dermal cylindroma and eccrine spiradenoma. *Australas J Dermatol* 1996;37:48–9.

Soyer PH, Rigel DS, Wurm EMT. Actinic keratosis, basal cell carcinoma and squamous cell carcinoma. In: Bolognia J, Jorizzo J, Schaffer J (eds) *Dermatology* 3e. St Louis: Elsevier Saunders 2012: 1845

APOCRINE HIDROCYSTOMA

Barnhill R, Crowson AN, Magro CM, Piepkorn MW. In *Dermatopathology*. New York: McGraw-Hill; 2010: 756–7

Sarabi K, Khachemoune A. Hidrocystomas: A brief review. *MedGenMed* 2006;8:57.

Stone M. Cysts. In: In: Bolognia J, Jorizzo J, Schaffer J (eds) *Dermatology* 3e. St Louis: Elsevier Saunders 2012: 1823–4.

Verma SB. Multiple apocrine hidrocystomas: A confusing clinical diagnosis. *An Bras Dermatol* 2010;85:260–3.

Wolff K, Johnson RA, Fitzpatrick TB. Hidrocystoma. In: *Fitzpatrick's Color Atlas and Synopsis of Clinical Dermatology*. New York: McGraw-Hill; 2009: 1070.

MIXED TUMOR

Barnhill R, Crowson AN, Magro CM, Piepkorn MW. In *Dermatopathology*. New York: McGraw-Hill; 2010: 735-7

McCalmont T. Adnexal neoplasms. In Bolognia J, Jorizzo J, Schaffer J (eds) *Dermatology* 3e. Philadelphia: Elsevier/ Saunders; 2012: 1831-4

Tirumalae R, Boer Almut. Calcification and ossification in eccrine mixed tumors: Underrecognized feature and diagnostic pitfall. *Am J Dermatopathol* 2009; 31:772–7.

Yavuzer R, Baŏterzi Y, Sari A, Bir F, Sezer C. Chondroid syringoma: a diagnosis more frequent than expected. *Dermatol Surg* 2003;29:179–81.

SPIRADENOMA

Barnhill R, Crowson AN, Magro CM, Piepkorn MW. In *Dermatopathology*. New York: McGraw-Hill; 2010: 725-6.

Elder D, Elenitsas R, Ragsdale BD. Tumors of the epidermal appendages. In: Elder D, Elenitas R, Jaworsky C, Johnson B (eds) *Lever's Histopathology of the Skin* 8e. Philadelphia: Lippincott-Raven; 1997: 888-90.

Johnston RB. *Weedon's Skin Pathology Essentials*. Edinburgh: Elsevier/Churchill Livingstone; 2012: 595.

McCalmont T. Adnexal neoplasms. In Bolognia J, Jorizzo J, Schaffer J (eds) *Dermatology* 3e. Philadelphia: Elsevier/ Saunders; 2012: 1844-5

Wolff K, Johnson RA, Fitzpatrick TB. Epidermal and appendageal tumors; Appendage tumors and hamartomas of the skin. In: *Fitzpatrick's Color Atlas and Synopsis of Clinical Dermatology*. New York: McGraw-Hill; 2009: 1076, 1079.

SYRINGOMA

Barnhill R, Crowson AN, Magro CM, Piepkorn MW. In *Dermatopathology*. New York: McGraw-Hill; 2010: 726–8.

McCalmont T. Adnexal neoplasms. In Bolognia J, Jorizzo J, Schaffer J (eds) *Dermatology* 3e. Philadelphia: Elsevier/Saunders; 2012: 1841.

POROMA

Barnhill R, Crowson AN, Magro CM, Piepkorn MW. In *Dermatopathology*. New York: McGraw-Hill; 2010: 728–30.

Harvell JD, Kerschmann RL, LeBoit PE. Eccrine or apocrine poroma? Six poromas with divergent adnexal differentiation. *Am J Dermatopathol* 1996;18:1–9.

McCalmont TH. A call for logic in the classification of adnexal neoplasms. *Am J Dermatopathol* 1996;18:103–9.

ADENOID CYSTIC CARCINOMA

Barnhill R, Crowson AN, Magro CM, Piepkorn MW. In *Dermatopathology*. New York: McGraw-Hill; 2010: 741.

Elder D, Elenitsas R, Ragsdale BD. Tumors of the epidermal appendages. In: Elder D, Elenitas R, Jaworsky C, Johnson B (eds) *Lever's Histopathology of the Skin* 8e. Philadelphia: Lippincott-Raven; 1997: 899

Rigel DS. Adnexal cancers of the skin. In: *Cancer of the Skin*. Philadelphia: Elsevier/Saunders; 2005: 297.

Weedon D. *Weedon's Skin Pathology* 3e. Edinburgh: Elsevier/Churchill Livingstone; 2010: 790.

MICROCYSTIC ADNEXAL CARCINOMA

McCalmont T. Adnexal neoplasms. In Bolognia J, Jorizzo J, Schaffer J (eds) *Dermatology* 3e. Philadelphia: Elsevier/Saunders; 2012: 1846.

Johnston RB. *Weedon's Skin Pathology Essentials*. Edinburgh: Elsevier/Churchill Livingstone; 2012: 605.

Elston D, Ferringer T. *Requisites in Dermatology. Dermatopathology*. Philadelphia: Elsevier/Saunders; 2009: 92–3.

EXTRAMAMMARY PAGET'S DISEASE

Villada G, Farooq U, Yu W, Diaz JP, Milikowski C. Extramammary Paget diseaseof the vulva with underlying mammary-like lobular carcinoma: A case report and review of the literature. *Am J Dermatopathol* 2014 April 17; [Epub ahead of print].

LeBoit PE, Burg G, Weedon D, Sarasin A (eds). *Pathology and Genetics of Skin Tumors*. Lyon: IARC Press; 2006: 136–8.

HIDRADENOCARCINOMA

Barnhill RL, Crowson AN (eds). *Textbook of Dermato*pathology 2e. New York: McGraw-Hill 2004: 739-40.

Johnston RB. *Weedon's Skin Pathology Essentials*. Edinburgh: Elsevier/Churchill Livingstone; 2012: 598.

Ko CJ, Cochran AJ, Eng W, et al. Hidradenocarcinoma: a histological and immunohistochemical study. *J Cutan Pathol* 2006;33:726–30.

Ohta M, Hiramoto M, Fujii M, Togo T. Nodular hidradrenocarcinoma on the scalp of a young woman: case report and review of lecture. *Dermatol Surg* 2004;30: 1265–8.

Weedon D. *Weedon's Skin Pathology* 3e. Edinburgh: Elsevier/Churchill Livingstone; 2010: 791-2.

POROCARCINOMA

Nguyen A, Nguyen AV. Eccrine porocarcinoma: a report of 2 cases and review of the literature. *Cutis* 2014;93:43–6.

Robson A, Greene J, Ansari N, et al. Eccrine porocarcinoma (malignant eccrine poroma): a clinicopathologic study of 69 cases. *Am J Surg Pathol* 2001;25:710–20.

4 TUMORS OF FIBROUS TISSUE

NODULAR FASCIITIS

Bolognia J, Jorizzo J, Schaffer J (eds) *Dermatology 3e. Philadelphia: Elsevier/Saunders 2012.*

Fletcher CDM, Unni KK, Mertens F. Pathology and Genetics of Tumours of Soft Tissue and Bone. Lyon: IARC Press; 2002.

LeBoit PE, Burg G, Weedon D, Sarasin A. Pathology and Genetics of Skin Tumours. Lyon: IARC Press; 2006.

Rapini R. Practical Dermatopathology. Philadelphia: Elsevier/Mosby; 2005.

Weedon D. Skin Pathology 2e. Edinburgh: Elsevier/Churchill Livingstone; 2002.

DERMATOFIBROMA

Chen TC, Kuo T, Chan HL. Dermatofibroma is a clonal proliferative disease. *J Cutan Pathol* 2000;27:36–9.

Granter, SR., Folpe, AL. Fibrous and fibrohistiocytic tumors. In: Barnhill, RL, Crowson, NA. Textbook of Dermatopathology 2e. New York: McGraw-Hill; 2004: 794–8.

Samlaska C, Bennion S. Eruptive dermatofibromas in a kindred. Cutis 2002;69:187–8, 190.

Weedon D. Weedon's Skin Pathology 3e. Edinburgh: Elsevier/Churchill Livingstone; 2010: 827–32.

Zaballos P, Puig S, Llambrich A, Malvehy J. Dermoscopy of dermatofibromas: a prospective morphological study of 412 cases. Arch Dermatol 2008;144:75–83.

SUPERFICIAL FIBROMATOSIS

Calonje E, Brenn T, Lazar A, McKee PH. McKee's Pathology of the Skin with Clinical Correlations, 4e. Edinburgh: Elsevier/Saunders; 2012.

Rapini R. Practical Dermatopathology. Philadelphia: Elsevier/Mosby; 2005.

Weedon D. Skin Pathology 2e. Edinburgh: Elsevier/Churchill Livingstone; 2002.

FIBROSARCOMAS

Bolognia, JL, Jorizzo, JL (eds). *Dermatology 2e. Philadelphia: Elsevier/Saunders; 2007.*

Fletcher CDM, Unni KK, Mertens F. *Pathology and Genetics of Tumours of Soft Tissue and Bone. Lyon: IARC Press; 2002.*

Weedon D. *Skin Pathology 2e. Edinburgh: Elsevier/Churchill Livingstone; 2002.*

DERMATOFIBROSARCOMA PROTUBERANS

Bolognia J, Jorizzo J, Schaffer J (eds) *Dermatology 3e. Philadelphia: Elsevier/Saunders 2012.*

Fletcher CDM, Unni KK, Mertens F. *Pathology and Genetics of Tumours of Soft Tissue and Bone. Lyon: IARC Press; 2002.*

LeBoit PE, Burg G, Weedon D, Sarasin A. *Pathology and Genetics of Skin Tumours. Lyon: IARC Press; 2006.*

Rapini R. *Practical Dermatopathology. Philadelphia: Elsevier/Mosby; 2005.*

Weedon D. *Skin Pathology 2e. Edinburgh: Elsevier/Churchill Livingstone; 2002.*

ATYPICAL FIBROXANTHOMA

Bolognia J, Jorizzo J, Schaffer J (eds) *Dermatology 3e. Philadelphia: Elsevier/Saunders 2012.*

Fletcher CDM, Unni KK, Mertens F. *Pathology and Genetics of Tumours of Soft Tissue and Bone. Lyon: IARC Press; 2002.*

LeBoit PE, Burg G, Weedon D, Sarasin A. *Pathology and Genetics of Skin Tumours. Lyon: IARC Press; 2006.*

Rapini R. *Practical Dermatopathology. Philadelphia: Elsevier/Mosby; 2005.*

Weedon D. *Skin Pathology 2e. Edinburgh: Elsevier/Churchill Livingstone; 2002.*

5 TUMORS OF FAT

LIPOMA

Calonje E, Brenn T, Lazar A, McKee PH. *McKee's Pathology of the Skin with Clinical Correlations, 4e. Edinburgh: Elsevier/Saunders; 2012.*

Weedon D. *Skin Pathology 2e. Edinburgh: Elsevier/Churchill Livingstone; 2002.*

ANGIOLIPOMA

Barnhill RL, Crowson AN, Magro CM, Piepkorn MW (eds). *Dermatopathology 3e. New York: McGraw-Hill; 2010: 858–9.*

Weedon D. *Weedon's Skin Pathology 3e. Edinburgh: Elsevier/Churchill Livingstone; 2010: 849–50.*

NEVUS LIPOMATOSUS SUPERFICIALIS

Bolognia J, Jorizzo J, Schaffer J (eds) *Dermatology 3e. Philadelphia: Elsevier/Saunders 2012.*

Calonje E, Brenn T, Lazar A, McKee PH. *McKee's Pathology of the Skin with Clinical Correlations, 4e. Edinburgh: Elsevier/Saunders; 2012.*

Weedon D. *Skin Pathology 2e. Edinburgh: Elsevier/Churchill Livingstone; 2002.*

6 TUMORS OF SMOOTH MUSCLE

LEIOMYOMA

Barnhill RL. Neoplasias and hyperplasias of muscular and neural origin. In *Dermatopathology. New York: McGraw-Hill Medical; 2010: 1172–3.*

Kohler, S. Muscle, Adipose and cartilage neoplasms. In: Bolognia J, Jorizzo JL, Rapini, RP (eds) *Dermatology 2e. St. Louis: Elsevier/Mosby; 2008: 1831–3.*

Wolff K, Goldsmith LA, Katz SI, Gilchrest BA, Paller AS, Leffell DJ. Tumors of muscle. In *Fitzpatrick's Dermatology in General Medicine. New York: McGraw-Hill Medical 2008: 868–70.*

LEIOMYOSARCOMA

Bolognia J, Jorizzo J, Schaffer J (eds) *Dermatology 3e. Philadelphia: Elsevier/Saunders 2012.*

Weedon D. *Skin Pathology 2e. Edinburgh: Elsevier/Churchill Livingstone; 2002.*

Calonje E, Brenn T, Lazar A, McKee PH. *McKee's Pathology of the Skin with Clinical Correlations, 4e. Edinburgh: Elsevier/Saunders; 2012.*

7 NEURAL TUMORS

NEUROFIBROMA

Bolognia J, Jorizzo J, Schaffer J (eds) *Dermatology 3e. Philadelphia: Elsevier/Saunders 2012.*

Calonje E, Brenn T, Lazar A, McKee PH. *McKee's Pathology of the Skin with Clinical Correlations, 4e. Edinburgh: Elsevier/Saunders; 2012.*

Elder D, Elenitsas R, Jaworsky C, Johnson Jr B. Neurofibromas (hamartomas with phenotypic diversity). In: *Lever's Histopathology of the Skin 8e. Philadelphia: Lippincott-Raven; 1997: 978*

Habif TP. Neurofibromatosis. In: *Clinical Dermatology. Philadelphia: Elsevier/Mosby; 2004: 905–8.*

Weedon D. *Skin Pathology 2e. Edinburgh: Elsevier/Churchill Livingstone; 2002.*

SCHWANNOMA

Bolognia J, Jorizzo J, Schaffer J (eds) *Dermatology 3e. Philadelphia: Elsevier/Saunders 2012.*

Calonje E, Brenn T, Lazar A, McKee PH. *McKee's Pathology of the Skin with Clinical Correlations, 4e. Edinburgh: Elsevier/Saunders; 2012.*

Weedon D. *Skin Pathology 2e. Edinburgh: Elsevier/Churchill Livingstone; 2002.*

PERINEURIOMA

Bolognia J, Jorizzo J, Schaffer J (eds) *Dermatology 3e. Philadelphia: Elsevier/Saunders 2012.*

Calonje E, Brenn T, Lazar A, McKee PH. *McKee's Pathology of the Skin with Clinical Correlations, 4e.* Edinburgh: Elsevier/ Saunders; 2012.

Fletcher CDM, Unni KK, Mertens F. *Pathology and Genetics of Tumours of Soft Tissue and Bone.* Lyon: IARC Press; 2002.

Weedon D. *Skin Pathology 2e.* Edinburgh: Elsevier/Churchill Livingstone; 2002.

PALISADED AND ENCAPSULATED NEUROMAS

Bolognia J, Jorizzo J, Schaffer J (eds) *Dermatology 3e.* Philadelphia: Elsevier/Saunders 2012.

Calonje E, Brenn T, Lazar A, McKee PH. *McKee's Pathology of the Skin with Clinical Correlations, 4e.* Edinburgh: Elsevier/ Saunders; 2012.

Fletcher CDM, Unni KK, Mertens F. *Pathology and Genetics of Tumours of Soft Tissue and Bone.* Lyon: IARC Press; 2002.

Weedon D. *Skin Pathology 2e.* Edinburgh: Elsevier/Churchill Livingstone; 2002.

CUTANEOUS GANGLIONEUROMA

Bolognia J, Jorizzo J, Schaffer J (eds) *Dermatology 3e.* Philadelphia: Elsevier/Saunders 2012.

Calonje E, Brenn T, Lazar A, McKee PH. *McKee's Pathology of the Skin with Clinical Correlations, 4e.* Edinburgh: Elsevier/ Saunders; 2012.

Fletcher CDM, Unni KK, Mertens F. *Pathology and Genetics of Tumours of Soft Tissue and Bone.* Lyon: IARC Press; 2002.

Weedon D. *Skin Pathology 2e.* Edinburgh: Elsevier/Churchill Livingstone; 2002.

NASAL GLIOMA

Bolognia J, Jorizzo J, Schaffer J (eds) *Dermatology 3e.* Philadelphia: Elsevier/Saunders 2012.

Calonje E, Brenn T, Lazar A, McKee PH. *McKee's Pathology of the Skin with Clinical Correlations, 4e.* Edinburgh: Elsevier/ Saunders; 2012.

Fletcher CDM, Unni KK, Mertens F. *Pathology and Genetics of Tumours of Soft Tissue and Bone.* Lyon: IARC Press; 2002.

Weedon D. *Skin Pathology 2e.* Edinburgh: Elsevier/Churchill Livingstone; 2002.

CUTANEOUS MENINGIOMA

Bolognia J, Jorizzo J, Schaffer J (eds) *Dermatology 3e.* Philadelphia: Elsevier/Saunders 2012.

Calonje E, Brenn T, Lazar A, McKee PH. *McKee's Pathology of the Skin with Clinical Correlations, 4e.* Edinburgh: Elsevier/ Saunders; 2012.

Fletcher CDM, Unni KK, Mertens F. *Pathology and Genetics of Tumours of Soft Tissue and Bone.* Lyon: IARC Press; 2002.

Weedon D. *Skin Pathology 2e.* Edinburgh: Elsevier/Churchill Livingstone; 2002.

GRANULAR CELL TUMOR

Bolognia J, Jorizzo J, Schaffer J (eds) *Dermatology 3e.* Philadelphia: Elsevier/Saunders 2012.

Calonje E, Brenn T, Lazar A, McKee PH. *McKee's Pathology of the Skin with Clinical Correlations, 4e.* Edinburgh: Elsevier/ Saunders; 2012.

Fletcher CDM, Unni KK, Mertens F. *Pathology and Genetics of Tumours of Soft Tissue and Bone.* Lyon: IARC Press; 2002.

Weedon D. *Skin Pathology 2e.* Edinburgh: Elsevier/Churchill Livingstone; 2002.

8 VASCULAR TUMORS

PYOGENIC GRANULOMA

Johnston RB. *Weedon's Skin Pathology Essentials.* Edinburgh: Elsevier/Churchill Livingstone; 2012: 704.

North PE, Kincannon J. Vascular neoplasms and neoplastic-like proliferations. In: Bolognia J, Jorizzo J, Schaffer J. *Dermatology (eds) Dermatology 3e.* Philadelphia: Elsevier/ Saunders 2012: 1922–3.

INFANTILE HEMANGIOMAS

Johnston RB. *Weedon's Skin Pathology Essentials.* Edinburgh: Elsevier/Churchill Livingstone; 2012: 594.

Kempf W, Hantschke M, Kutzner H, Burgdorf W. *Dermatopathology.* New York: Springer; 2008:262–3.

Sangueza OP, Requena L. *Pathology of Vascular Skin Lesions: Clinicopathologic Correlations.* New York: Humana Press; 2003: 136–50.

CHERRY ANGIOMAS

Sangueza OP, Requena L. *Pathology of Vascular Skin Lesions: Clinicopathologic Correlations.* New York: Humana Press; 2003: 151–3.

ARTERIOVENOUS HEMANGIOMA

Sangueza OP, Requena L. *Pathology of Vascular Skin Lesions: Clinicopathologic Correlations.* New York: Humana Press; 2003: 154–6.

MICROVENULAR HEMANGIOMA

Sangueza OP, Requena L. *Pathology of Vascular Skin Lesions: Clinicopathologic Correlations.* New York: Humana Press; 2003: 161–3.

TUFTED ANGIOMA

Sangueza OP, Requena L. *Pathology of Vascular Skin Lesions: Clinicopathologic Correlations.* New York: Humana Press; 2003: 164–8.

GLOMERULOID HEMANGIOMA

Sangueza OP, Requena L. *Pathology of Vascular Skin Lesions: Clinicopathologic Correlations.* New York: Humana Press; 2003: 169–73.

Acquired elastotic hemangioma

Sangueza OP, Requena L. Pathology of Vascular Skin Lesions: Clinicopathologic Correlations. New York: Humana Press; 2003: 174–76.

Kaposiform hemangioendothelioma

Sangueza OP, Requena L. Pathology of Vascular Skin Lesions: Clinicopathologic Correlations. New York: Humana Press; 2003: 177–81.

Glomus tumor and glomangioma

Johnston RB. *Weedon's Skin Pathology Essentials.* Edinburgh: Elsevier/Churchill Livingstone; 2012: 707.

North PE, Kincannon J. Vascular neoplasms and neoplastic-like proliferations. In: Bolognia J, Jorizzo J, Schaffer J. Dermatology (eds) Dermatology 3e. Philadelphia: Elsevier/ Saunders 2012: 1937–9.

Kaposi's sarcoma

Johnston RB. *Weedon's Skin Pathology Essentials.* Edinburgh: Elsevier/Churchill Livingstone; 2012: 712.

North PE, Kincannon J. Vascular neoplasms and neoplastic-like proliferations. In: Bolognia J, Jorizzo J, Schaffer J. Dermatology (eds) Dermatology 3e. Philadelphia: Elsevier/ Saunders 2012: 1932–5.

Angiosarcoma

Johnston RB. *Weedon's Skin Pathology Essentials.* Edinburgh: Elsevier/Churchill Livingstone; 2012: 714.

North PE, Kincannon J. Vascular neoplasms and neoplastic-like proliferations. In: Bolognia J, Jorizzo J, Schaffer J. Dermatology (eds) Dermatology 3e. Philadelphia: Elsevier/ Saunders 2012: 1935–6.

9 Cutaneous Cysts

Epidermoid cyst

Barnhill RL, Crowson AN (eds). *Textbook of Dermatopathology 2e. New York: McGraw-Hill 2004: 563.*

Rapini R. *Practical Dermatopathology. St Louis: Elsevier/Mosby; 2005: 253.*

Stone MS. Cysts. In Bolognia J, Jorizzo J, Schaffer J. Dermatology 3e. Philadelphia: Elsevier/Saunders; 2012: 1817–23.

Wolff K, Johnson RA, Suurmond D. Fitzpatrick's Color Atlas and Synopsis of Clinical Dermatology 5e. New York: McGraw-Hill; 2005: 199.

Pilar cyst

Alsaad KO, Obaidat NA, Ghazarian D. Skin adnexal neoplasms–part 1: an approach to tumours of the pilosebaceous unit. *J Clin Pathol* 2007;60:129–44.

Barnhill RL, Crowson AN (eds). Textbook of Dermatopathology 3e. New York: McGraw-Hill 2010: 544.

Fernández-Figueras MT, Casalots A, Puig L, Llatjós R, Ferrándiz C, Ariza A. Proliferating trichilemmal tumour: p53 immunoreactivity in association with p27Kip1 over-expression indicates a low-grade carcinoma profile. *Histopathology* 2001;38:454–7.

Dermoid cyst

Barnhill RL, Crowson AN (eds). *Textbook of Dermatopathology 2e. New York: McGraw-Hill 2004: 564–7.*

Rapini R. *Practical Dermatopathology. St Louis: Elsevier/Mosby; 2005: 253–5.*

Stone MS. Cysts. In Bolognia J, Jorizzo J, Schaffer J. Dermatology 3e. Philadelphia: Elsevier/Saunders; 2012: 1822–3.

Wolff K, Johnson RA, Suurmond D. Fitzpatrick's Color Atlas and Synopsis of Clinical Dermatology 5e. New York: McGraw-Hill; 2005.

Steatocystoma

Barnhill RL, Crowson AN (eds). *Textbook of Dermatopathology 2e. New York: McGraw-Hill 2004: 563–7.*

Rapini R. *Practical Dermatopathology. St Louis: Elsevier/Mosby; 2005: 255–6.*

Stone MS. Cysts. In Bolognia J, Jorizzo J, Schaffer J. Dermatology 3e. Philadelphia: Elsevier/Saunders; 2012: 1821–2.

Wolff K, Johnson RA, Suurmond D. Fitzpatrick's Color Atlas and Synopsis of Clinical Dermatology 5e. New York: McGraw-Hill; 2005.

Bronchogenic cyst

Barnhill RL, Crowson AN (eds). *Textbook of Dermatopathology 2e. New York: McGraw-Hill 2004: 564–8.*

Rapini R. *Practical Dermatopathology. St Louis: Elsevier/Mosby; 2005.*

Stone MS. Cysts. In Bolognia J, Jorizzo J, Schaffer J. Dermatology 3e. Philadelphia: Elsevier/Saunders; 2012: 1824.

Wolff K, Johnson RA, Suurmond D. Fitzpatrick's Color Atlas and Synopsis of Clinical Dermatology 5e. New York: McGraw-Hill; 2005.

Cutaneous ciliated cyst

Barnhill RL, Crowson AN (eds). *Textbook of Dermatopathology 2e. New York: McGraw-Hill 2004: 564–9.*

Rapini R. *Practical Dermatopathology. St Louis: Elsevier/Mosby; 2005: 256.*

Stone MS. Cysts. In Bolognia J, Jorizzo J, Schaffer J. Dermatology 3e. Philadelphia: Elsevier/Saunders; 2012: 1825.

Wolff K, Johnson RA, Suurmond D. Fitzpatrick's Color Atlas and Synopsis of Clinical Dermatology 5e. New York: McGraw-Hill; 2005.

Median raphe cyst

Barnhill RL, Crowson AN (eds). *Textbook of Dermatopathology 2e. New York: McGraw-Hill 2004: 570.*

Rapini R. *Practical Dermatopathology. St Louis: Elsevier/Mosby; 2005: 259.*

Stone MS. Cysts. In Bolognia J, Jorizzo J, Schaffer J. *Dermatology 3e. Philadelphia: Elsevier/Saunders; 2012: 1824–5.*

Wolff K, Johnson RA, Suurmond D. *Fitzpatrick's Color Atlas and Synopsis of Clinical Dermatology 5e. New York: McGraw-Hill; 2005.*

10 CUTANEOUS METASTASES

Weedon D. *Weedon's Skin Pathology 3e. Edinburgh: Elsevier/Churchill Livingstone; 2010: 928–33.*

11 CUTANOUS INFILTRATES, NON LYMPHOID

MASTOCYTOSIS

Brockow K. Epidemiology, prognosis, and risk factors in mastocytosis. *Immunol Allergy Clin North Am 2014;34:283–95.*

Weedon D. *Weedon's Skin Pathology 3e. Edinburgh: Elsevier/Churchill Livingstone; 2010: 947–9.*

JUVENILE XANTHOGRANULOMA

Satter EK, Walters MC, Hurt M, Bolton JG, Dever T. A brief overview of the most common histiocytic disorders. *G Ital Dermatol Venereol 2010;145:717–31.*

Weedon D. *Weedon's Skin Pathology 3e. Edinburgh: Elsevier/Churchill Livingstone; 2010: 953–4.*

XANTHOMAS

Barnhill RL, Crowson AN, Magro CM, Piepkorn MW (eds). *Dermatopathology 3e. New York: McGraw-Hill; 2010:113–6.*

Fleischmajer R. Cutaneous and tendon xanthomas. *Dermatologica1964;128:113–32.*

Weedon D. *Weedon's Skin Pathology 3e. Edinburgh: Elsevier/Churchill Livingstone; 2010: 961–3.*

LANGERHANS CELL HISTIOCYTOSIS

Satter EK, Walters MC, Hurt M, Bolton JG, Dever T. A brief overview of the most common histiocytic disorders. *G Ital Dermatol Venereol 2010;145:717–31.*

Weedon D. *Weedon's Skin Pathology 3e. Edinburgh: Elsevier/Churchill Livingstone; 2010: 966–7.*

MERKEL CELL CARCINOMA

Kuwamoto S. Recent advances in the biology of Merkel cell carcinoma. *Hum Pathol 2011;42:1063–77.*

LeBoit PE, Burg G, Weedon D, Sarasin A (eds). *Pathology and Genetics of Skin Tumors. Lyon: IARC Press; 2006: 272–3.*

Succaria F, Radfar A, Bhawan J. Merkel cell carcinoma (primary neuroendocrine carcinoma of skin) mimicking basal cell carcinoma with review of different histopathologic features. *Am J Dermatopathol 2014;36:160–6.*

12 CUTANEOUS INFILTRATES, LYMPHOID AND LEUKEMIC

CUTANEOUS PSEUDOLYMPHOMAS (LYMPHOID HYPERPLASIA)

LeBoit PE, Burg G, Weedon D, Sarasain A (eds). *World Health Orgnization Classification of Tumors. Pathology and Genetics of Skin Tumors. Lyon: IARC Press; 2006: 213–4.*

Weedon D. *Weedon's Skin Pathology 3e. Edinburgh: Elsevier/Churchill Livingstone; 2010: 1000–2.*

T-CELL LYMPHOMAS

LeBoit PE, Burg G, Weedon D, Sarasain A (eds). *World Health Orgnization Classification of Tumors. Pathology and Genetics of Skin Tumors. Lyon: IARC Press; 2006: 170–91.*

Weedon D. *Weedon's Skin Pathology 3e. Edinburgh: Elsevier/Churchill Livingstone; 2010: 973–85.*

Primary cutaneous CD30+ T-cell lymphoproliferative disorders

Kunishige JH, McDonald H, Alvarez G, Johnson M, Prieto V, Duvic M. Lymphomatoid papulosis and associated lymphomas: a retrospective case series of 84 patients. *Clin Exp Dermatol 2009;34:576–81.*

McQuitty E, Curry JL, Tetzlaff MT, Prieto VG, Duvic M, Torres-Cabala C. The differential diagnosis of CD8-positive ("type D") lymphomatoid papulosis. J Cutan Pathol 2014;41:88–100.*

B-CELL LYMPHOMAS

LeBoit PE, Burg G, Weedon D, Sarasain A (eds). *World Health Orgnization Classification of Tumors. Pathology and Genetics of Skin Tumors. Lyon: IARC Press; 2006: 195–99.*

Weedon D. *Weedon's Skin Pathology 3e. Edinburgh: Elsevier/Churchill Livingstone; 2010: 987–91.*

LEUKEMIA CUTIS

LeBoit PE, Burg G, Weedon D, Sarasain A (eds). *World Health Orgnization Classification of Tumors. Pathology and Genetics of Skin Tumors. Lyon: IARC Press; 2006: 211.*

Weedon D. *Weedon's Skin Pathology 3e. Edinburgh: Elsevier/Churchill Livingstone; 2010: 996–9.*

GLOSSARY OF TERMS

EPIDERMAL

a. **Hyperkeratosis** - thickening of the stratum corneum

Hyperkeratosis

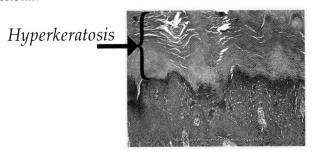

b. **Orthokeratosis** - 'basket-weave' appearance of the stratum corneum without retention of keratinocyte nuclei

Orthokeratosis

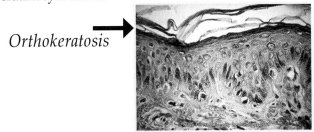

c. **Parakeratosis** - the retention of nuclei by keratinocytes in the stratum corneum

Column of parakera-tosis with surrounding ortho-keratosis

Ortho-keratosis

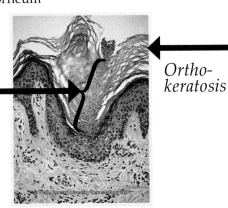

d. **Hypergranulosis** - increased granules in the keratinocytes of the stratum granulosum

Hypergranulosis

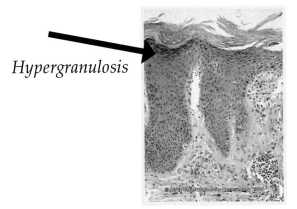

e. **Hypogranulosis** - decreased granules in the keratino-cytes of the stratum granulosum

Hypogranulosis

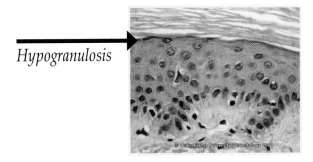

f. **Hyperplasia** - an increased number of cells
i. *Psoriasiform* - regular acanthosis with elongated rete ridges of the same length

Psoriasiform hyperplasia

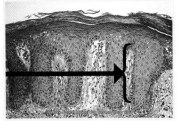

ii. *Irregular* - acanthosis with rete ridges of differing lengths, often pointed

Irregular hyperplasia with pointed rete ridges

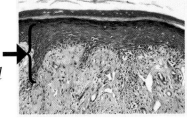

iii. *Papillated* - thickening of the epidermis with nipple-like elevations

Papillated hyperplasia

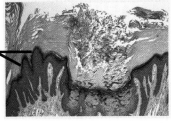

iv. *Pseudocarcinomatous* - extreme, irregular thicken-ing of the epidermis with increased mitoses, squamous eddies, or keratin pearls which may mimic squamous cell carcinoma.

Keratin pearl

Irregular epidermal hyperplasia

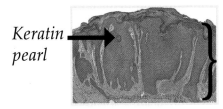

1. Squamous eddy - concentric, whorled groups of keratinocytes with increased keratinization towards the center

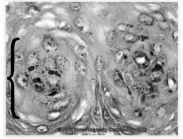

Squamous eddy

2. *Horn (or keratin) pearl* - a squamous eddy with more abrupt and complete keratinization

Keratin pearls

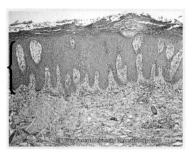

g. **Acanthosis** - diffuse epidermal hyperplasia, especially of the stratum spinosum

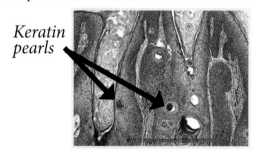

Acanthosis

h. **Atrophy** - decreased thickness of a tissue or layer

Epidermal atrophy with loss of rete ridges and dermal papilla pattern

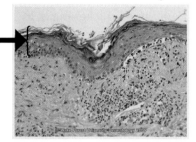

i. **Spongiosis** - intercellular edema expands the space between keratinocytes and can cause the cells to become elongated or stretched

Spongiosis and formation of intraepidermal vesicles

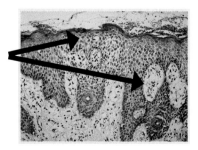

j. **Ballooning** - intracellular edema that eventually causes loss of attachment to adjacent cells (secondary acantholysis), generally due to viral particles

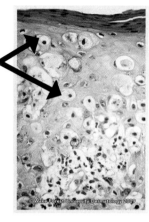

Ballooning degeneration of epidermal cells

k. **Acantholysis** - the loss of cohesion between keratinocytes due to dissolution of intercellular connections (desmosomes) (see **Dyskeratosis** photo)

l. **Spongiform pustule** - collections of neutrophils in the spinous layer

Spongiform pustules

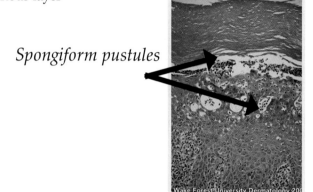

m. **Dyskeratosis** - abnormal or premature cornification of keratinocytes

Dyskeratosis
Acantholysis

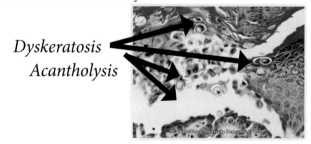

n. **Necrosis** - cell death with subsequent degeneration

Necrosis

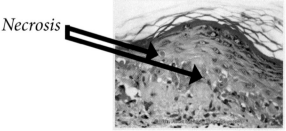

o. **Vacuolar alteration** - intracellular or extracellular clear space that causes damaged keratinocytes to appear vacuolated

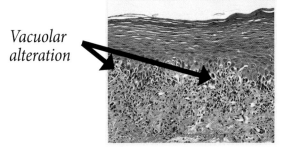

Vacuolar alteration

p. **Clefts** - an empty space, which may contain fluid, lipid, or other substances that is lost during tissue processing

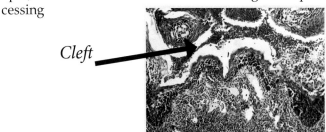

Cleft

q. **Interface dermatitis** - liquefactive degeneration of the basal cell layer at the interface between the epidermis and dermis with sparse inflammation

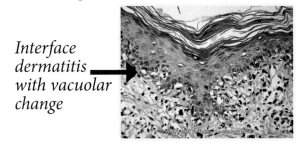

Interface dermatitis with vacuolar change

DERMAL

a. **Monomorphous infiltrate** - abnormal presence of inflammatory cells of one cell type

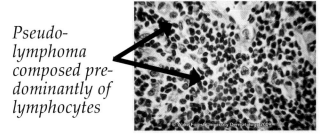

Pseudo-lymphoma composed predominantly of lymphocytes

b. **Mixed infiltrate** - abnormal presence of inflammatory cells of multiple cell types

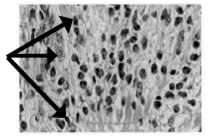

Mixed infiltrate of lymphocytes, histiocytes, and eosinophils in urticarial pemphigoid

c. **Lymphohistiocytic infiltrate**- a collection of lymphocytes and histiocytes

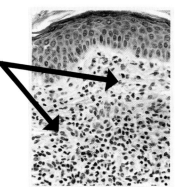

Mixed infiltrate of lymphocytes and histiocytes in pigmented purpuric dermatosis

d. **Lichenoid infiltrate** - a band-like configuration of inflammatory cells arranged parallel to the dermis

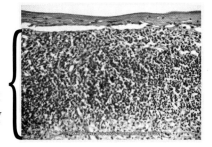

Band-like, lichenoid infiltrate seen in lichenoid drug reaction

e. **Nodular infiltrate** - dense discrete aggregations of inflammatory or tumor cells

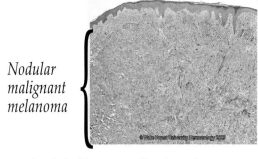

Nodular malignant melanoma

f. **Leukocytoclastic infiltrate** - collection of abnormal neutrophils characterized by chromatin fragmentation, nuclear dust, and necrotic debris

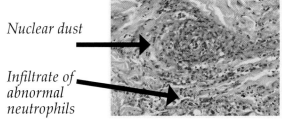

Nuclear dust

Infiltrate of abnormal neutrophils

g. **Diffuse infiltrate** - an infiltrate of inflammatory or tumor cells distributed in a nonlocalized fashion

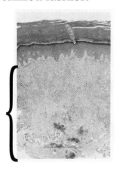

Diffuse infiltrate in superficial and deep dermis

123

Connective Tissue

a. **Collagen degeneration** - disorganized, fragmented mass of collagen (as opposed to the tightly packed, strictly aligned filaments normally seen)

Collagen degeneration alternating with areas of perivascular infiltrate

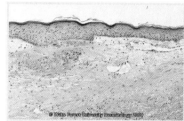

b. **Hyalinization of collagen** - relatively hypocellular, eosinophilic appearance of collagen

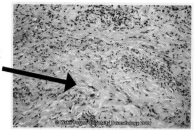

Hyalinized collagen with hypocellularity

More regular appearance of collagen compared to affected area above

c. **Fibrosis** - an increase in collagen associated with an increased number of fibroblasts

Increased collagen with an increased number of fibroblasts (at tip of lines)

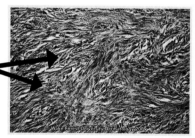

d. **Sclerosis** - an increase in collagen with either a normal or decreased number of fibroblasts

Thickened collagen throughout the dermis with decreased cellularity

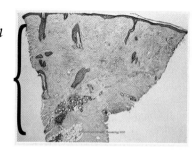

e. **Collagen in vertical streaks** - a vertical orientation of thick collagen bundles that occurs with chronic rubbing

Vertically streaked collagen within the papillary dermis

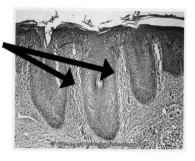

f. **Lamellated collagen** - layered, or plate-like arrangement of collagen

Whorls of layered collagen surrounding areas of increased melanocytes

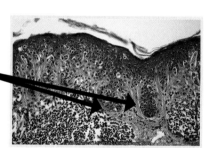